A Life In The Balance

By
Scott Burton

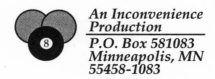

An Inconvenience Production
P.O. Box 581083
Minneapolis, MN
55458-1083

Many thanks to those who helped me put this book together:

Dr. Craig Hergert -- professor, writer, stand-up comic *and* fellow cancer survivor -- who not only served as editor but pushed me further and helped me become a better writer.

Marnie Deacon, who designed the cover -- thanks for your patience.

Thanks also to all those who supported me, read my endless revsions and are part of a larger group I consider myself fortunate to call friends. I wish I could list you all.

And my greatest thanks to my wife, without whose patience, sound advice and loving friendship I could have never completed this manuscript. She has not only been a great editor on all I've shown to her, but is also a great editor and counsel in my life.

This book is published by: *Inconvenience Productions*
P.O. Box 581083
Minneapolis, MN 55458-1083

This book is dedicated to Harvey Burton, 1920-1976

It is also dedicated to my wife, Cheryl, the unsung hero of my life.

With Love.

Contents

Introduction

My father passed away on July 19, 1996 from a metasticized melanoma. That was the second time cancer had struck my family. The first was when I battled an osteo sarcoma more than five years before he died. When he was first diagnosed, I simply assumed he would survive like I did. As his condition worsened and we realized that his survival was unlikely, I began to look more at the life he had led than at his dying.

I wasn't shocked nor did I fear for him even though I knew the pain I went through. In a strange way, I was proud of him. Dad responded to the call, not only facing cancer and his death, but of facing his life. I wanted to be around him while he did that and to remain a part of his life as long as I could. Although the disease ultimately took away his ability to recognize me, we sometimes were able to look at each other and laugh the way we used to before he had cancer.

By the time my father was diagnosed, I had been speaking about cancer for almost two years, hoping to help others facing cancer find joy in their lives even within their illnesses, even within their pain. I knew that in every discussion of cancer loomed the fear of death, but rarely did it also include the miracle of life. As my father passed away, I got to see both.

Of the many ways there are to approach cancer, I see two as being the most important. Many people are raising funds, doing research and everything they can to stop the horrible disease. The world's ability to fight cancer and win would not be nearly as great without these people — most of us owe our lives to them, not only because they have cured many of us but because they have also taught us how to avoid cancer.

But I sometimes wonder if maybe it's not so important whether we cure cancer or not. It seems as if there will always be another disease to take its place — AIDS, diabetes, heart disease, and there are new ones being discovered every day. Maybe an even worse disease is the fear of cancer, the fear of any disease, the fear of not of death, but of life.

My desire, during my cancer, was to, like my father, answer the call — to laugh, smile and embrace life as long as possible. This story is how I tried to do that.

This book is for both the people who want to laugh and find joy in every situation in life, as well as those who are afraid of life. Being afraid of life is the real disease: And that one is curable.

*"It's all the same
to share the pain
with me."*

*from the song,
Me In Honey
by R.E.M.*

First, A Word About Juggling: Throwing Up Three, Catching Two

I first learned to juggle in the mid-seventies when I was twelve or thirteen. They were days of revolution; Nixon resigned, the Apollo space missions were exploring a new frontier and civil rights advocates were forging new freedoms. Perhaps it was in the air or perhaps it was simply nature taking its course, but as an adolescent I had my own version of rebellion. It wasn't that I caused trouble at school, wore outlandish clothes or went out looking for fights. I was a quiet rebel. My rebellion had more to do with wanting to be an independent thinker than thumbing my nose at society. I was still polite, did my work and listened to my parents, but no matter what I did, I made sure I did it my own way. The worst thing anybody could do to me at that time was label me. When people thought I was quiet, I'd be loud. If they thought I was nothing but a joker, I'd be thoughtful and reflective. Juggling was the ideal expression for my rebellion: It was something that didn't offend anyone else but still let me do my own thing.

My brother Jack taught me to juggle in our mother's apartment on Pillsbury Avenue in Minneapolis while our parents were separated. One day, while we were passing time watching TV and visiting, he amazed me by taking three of my mom's oranges and teaching himself to juggle. Actually I was equally amazed that he even *wanted* to. "Why juggling?" I thought. "Isn't that for clowns?"

Why not shooting baskets as we often did, or going for a run or, my favorite pastime, sitting down and watching TV? For some reason, I still thought Jack's juggling was cool.

After he taught me the basics, I immediately saw the endless possibilities in juggling. Before I could even control the oranges, I envisioned tricks that I wanted to do once I could hold the basic pattern. Practicing all that summer in our living room, my independent side showed through. What also came through were the personal qualities that made me like every other juggler on the planet — a perfectionist's eye and an obsessive nature. Neither of us could have known that ten minutes with three oranges would lay the groundwork for my career, my personality and a major part of my life.

Although I embraced it more, Jack should have been the juggler in our family. With his desire to teach himself and his creativity, he would have been a wonderful juggler. But, alas, Jack had a life. He was a popular kid at school, had a tight group of friends and plenty of other things to do. I, on the other hand, had disconnected myself from any friends I might have had. Not at all prepared to handle the dynamics of social politics, especially at the cut-throat junior high level, I kept to myself, walking the halls in anonymity and preferring it that way. Although I was involved in sports, wrestling in particular, I didn't feel like I related well to the other kids my age. Besides, at school, I was intimidated by the teachers, the hallways and the boys smoking in the bathroom. In addition, I was in awe of the junior high girls who were turning into women. But whereas being socially inept is a curse for most adolescents, for a juggler it's nearly a requirement.

With my eagerness to improve and a near-lethal amount of free time, I surpassed Jack. I joined a juggler's group that practiced every Wednesday at a small park shelter. Although all of us in that group were socially dysfunctional, craved attention, and had sessions that would now be considered therapy, we had a strong sense of camaraderie and a commitment to juggling as an art.

Juggling had taken me many places. Although I had learned all my skills while practicing alone, once I joined a street theater group in Minneapolis called Sideshow, with other jugglers, storytellers and mimes, juggling had offically become my trade. I was leery at first, having felt that jugglers, computer geeks and Star Trek fans had all pretty much come from the same gene pool — the type of people that do something strangely unique, yet all seem to have the same personality. (If not for the obvious communication problem, mimes would be included as well.) But the people at Sideshow were down-to-earth normal people who simply enjoyed entertaining. With them I travelled throughout the Midwest performing at festivals and fairs. With them I cut my teeth in the performing world, going down to the Kansas City Renaissance Festival five years in a row. I moved on, after the fifth year, concluding that every man comes to a point in his life where he outgrows wearing tights.

I finally brought my act indoors, doing a solo show in comedy clubs. Around that time I met Cheryl, courted her as we rode around town on my motorcycle and, in May of 1985, married her. Juggling and comedy was my career until something better or at least more normal were to come along. But nothing ever did. Eventually I began doing corporate shows for executives and as after-dinner entertainment. The next thing we knew, Cheryl and I had bought a house, were raising our two children, Rachel and Dylan, and even saving a little money — all on a juggler's salary.

Because it's my nature to look on the opposite side of things, I kept thinking that, since everything was going so well, something also was bound to go wrong. And, in accordance with the laws of self-fulfilling prophecy, something did. Ten years after I started my juggling career, a year before being diagnosed with cancer and the same year we were expecting our third child, Matthew, something happened that shook my career as well as my perspective on life. It was the moment when I could no longer think of myself as a serious juggler.

Nearly a year before my diagnosis of cancer I was at a juggling competition. I remember feeling the pressure as I wandered backstage along with the seven other jugglers who were wearing smart outfits of sequined flash or vaudevillian style. One juggler rapidly threw seven balls into the air, catching them without a flaw. Another kept five clubs afloat while passing several behind his back. Yet another was fumbling with one ball, a hat and a small stool. Backstage had the feel of a showcase performance at a Vegas casino. But the glitz, scantily clad showgirls and cheap breakfast buffets were conspicuously absent. It wasn't Las Vegas. It was a small gym in St. Louis at a college where the 1991 International Juggler's Association convention was being held. That Friday night were the U.S. Nationals, and I was competing with the other jugglers who passed the qualifying round. After months of hard work, I had my sights set on a gold medal.

The show I made my living at was a comedy show, a blend of high-energy, stand-up comedy and playful juggling, but every so often I traveled to an IJA convention to try my hand at straight technical juggling to seven minutes of music. Having competed before, once winning the teams event with my good friend and juggling partner Bryan Wendling, once placing second in the U.S. Nationals, I had the feeling that this year was going to be the biggest one of them all. I was confident that I had come to the convention with juggling unlike anyone else was doing. For the previous year, almost two, I had been trying to figure out a new way to juggle, spending two to three hours a day in the basement of a warehouse in downtown Minneapolis. I tried inventing an unusual but athletic routine using only one club. I tried to come up with a routine with my back completely to the audience and all the action going on behind me. I tried to think of any trick that didn't look at all like what other jugglers were doing. Finally I came up with a routine that used asymetrical tricks and quarter turns so that half my tricks would be done as I was turned away from the audience.

It had always been my aim to juggle differently. Because I mostly practiced alone that wasn't hard to do, and the first routine I'd ever created was physical and made up of original tricks. My goal was to go from trick to trick without a rest so that even a juggler couldn't tell where one trick stopped and another started. A throw from behind my back would immediately go over my shoulder and then under my leg, and then I'd spin and catch it. While other jugglers highlighted the beauty of juggling, making their routines an elegant, whimsical dance, mine was a sock hop, a jitterbug marathon where anything goes. I preferred to juggle ugly. And with the new routine, I had taken it even further, adding a lot more unusual moves as well as a routine of rolls, kicks and odd throws while lying on my back.

Standing quietly backstage with the other guys I noticed that even my attire didn't fit the standard juggler mold. Wearing an all black outfit, garage sale tank top, cut-off shorts and vinyl shoes, I may have made Mike Tyson's best dressed list, but I sure didn't look like any of them. All the other guys looked like they were there to perform. They were showmen, a cross between David Copperfield and a used car salesman. I looked like I was there to clean up after the show. Part of me knew it was by choice. I do my comedy show to entertain the audience; my juggling routine I do for me. What I wear isn't important because I'm not entertaining but, rather, trying to let the juggling speak for itself. But, while part of me knew it was about juggling, the other part simply wanted recognition. I'd worked hard to be as good as I was and, even though I'd placed in previous competions, I still felt the way I did in junior high — intimidated by everyone else who seemed to know what they were doing. I still was out of the loop in the juggling world — and my style did not have wide acceptance.

Actually, I was out of the loop in more ways than one. Even on a personal level I didn't match up too well with other jugglers. Nowhere was that more apparent than at a convention where many jugglers used their art as their philosophical and metaphysical statements, turning their lives into an eternal roadshow. While there are many creative individuals and charming personalities at the conventions I attended, there were also the jugglers who seemed to act like all other jugglers. I remember once listening to a fellow

wearing a belled jester's hat and a goatee telling me that, "Juggling helps blend my physical and mental consciousness so I'm freer to communicate and more in touch with nature." I interpreted that to mean, "It keeps me from getting a real job, I like showing off, and I can do it naked. While I love juggling, embrace it as a living and use it as my art, I've tried never to lose sight of the fact that seals can do it.

With the attitude I brought to St. Louis, I may have set myself up for things to go wrong. Not relating completely on a personal level, entertaining in the same fasion or even stylistically fitting in, I somehow expected the room of 500 jugglers to immediately be taken with my new routine. I don't know what I was thinking. I knew it was good and I believed in it completely, but to think that a roomful of hardcore jugglers would be blown away by what might even be considered anti-juggling, was near delusional. Somehow it got to be less about the juggling and more about me. Whether I got along with the mainstream juggling world or not, I was hoping for recognition. It's like on the outside I was friendly and humble, just happy to be at the convention — but on the inside I was Vincent Price in a B-movie, "They all laughed at me at the college. But wait until they see what my death ray has in store for them. Ha ha ha ha."

The one thing I didn't expect, after having practiced my routine for nearly six months and thinking I would be a big hit at the convention, was the apocalyptic case of nerves I got once I reached St. Louis. It was amazing and I had never before felt anything quite like it. Yet the signs of my impending doom began popping up all over the place. In the cramped practice gym, with a hundred other jugglers, I couldn't focus on any of their routines much less my own. I was sweating so much that, after half an hour, the salty water ran down my arms, making my hands stick to my clubs. In addition, I was having trouble sleeping, had a terrible appetite and felt disoriented. I felt as if nothing was going right. Throughout the week I was unfocused and unhealthy and I didn't even know it meant I was scared; I thought the tension was adrenaline. The fact that my nerves were shot was obvious to an outsider but I didn't notice. Somehow I assumed I'd pull it all together by show time. Finally, at the rehearsal before the show, I was juggling three clubs in one hand. I threw two up and spun around attempting to catch them when one hit me squarely on my left eye. Although I finished the routine, blood was draining from a cut above my eye throughout dinner. That was when even I knew my nerves and ability had left for good. But I was scheduled to go on so, confident or not, I was determined to compete.

So there I was — physically tired, suffering from loss of appetite, jittery, unfocused and bleeding from my eye — and I was preparing for a major performance in front of my peers. I should have withdrawn from the competition. But apparently I needed an act of God to make that point, a burning bush perhaps, Mohammed on the mountain, Buddha at the Lotus tree, or maybe just some Hari Krishna guy to smack me on the back of the head and say, "What are you, stupid?"

Not taking heed of the signs all around me, I went to the back of the gym where the other jugglers were warming up. When my name was called, I walked into the spotlight at the middle of the makeshift stage backdropped by a black curtain. The bad omens continued as the music started before I even reached center stage. The person running the music was supposed to wait until I was in position; then I would begin rolling one ball between my open hands in rhythm to the music, creating the illusion that the ball was appearing and disappearing. Because of the error, I had to catch up to get my routine even with the music and felt shaky as if I were going to drop at any point. Once I did drop, it was like a bad dream as I dropped consecutively again and again. And it didn't end. When I juggled on my back, the ball rolled away so I had to get up and chase it. When I did a spin, I spun too far and found myself looking at the curtain as the club hit the floor behind me. By the tenth drop, out of necessity, I decided that dropping wasn't so bad after all. I hoped the integrity of my style remained intact. I hoped, even if it was no longer about me, the physical and less poetic side of my expression came through. But I was losing my integrity as fast as a stuttering talk show host loses his. Then, in the middle of the routine, as everything was already going wrong, I fell — as in down. I wasn't proud of the performance in the first place, but actually hitting the floor was a new lesson in humility. A juggler falling down in the middle of a national competition is like famed tenor Luciano Pavarotti reaching the crescendo of his closing aria and then, accidentally, swallowing a trumpet. Before arriving in St. Louis, I could have never imagined the routine being that magnificently bad.

I was trying to make an impression on my peers, yet I only distanced myself further from them — all because I had to be different. Even before the competition, a young woman remarked that my routine would be just as good if I cut out half the tricks. "Less is more," she said, and I agreed. But I still went ahead with the non-stop bit I came to the convention with. To do any less, I thought, would make the routine less mine, though, after I was done, I would have been better off if the routine *was* less mine.

It's embarrassing to admit that what I saw as finally going wrong in my life was a juggling routine gone awry. But I learned weeks later that it wasn't just about an abysmal display of juggling. It wasn't the fact that I fell on stage that left an indelible mark on me. The fact that I couldn't do anything right made me feel as if I weren't a juggler anymore. Looking back, I see that routine, the fear and sickness beforehand and my hitting the floor as being the time I passed the peak in the arc of my life. I saw the unfantastic, unaccomplished, unimportant face of my existence. Life flew by me like a speeding train and I didn't even have the chance to look at it. It was like male menopause, like the fear of turning 40, like screaming downhill on a roller coaster, racing toward oblivion. I saw that I wasn't destined for juggling greatness or greatness of any kind. I was only a fragile, simple human facing the same fate billions had faced before me. It was perhaps the ugliest thing I ever had to face. Yet my biggest failure prepared me for real life, for things going wrong, for the cancer yet to come.

While it was happening, I didn't understand the meaning of my routine going so badly. After I finished, I went and sat with my friends in the bleachers by the side of the stage. They looked at me like my number had just come up in the draft. Having seen me work hard at it and demand perfection, they knew what I expected from my juggling. They had heard me say months earlier, "All I care about in the competition is that I don't embarrass myself." Looking at their gaping faces I smiled and said, more or less, "Man, I stunk." They smiled, and, since their routine hadn't gone well either, we spent the rest of the evening laughing, relieved and sickened. As soon as the competitions were over, I went back to my dorm room, fell asleep and didn't wake until noon the next day, catching up on all the sleep I hadn't gotten for the past week.

Strangely, the next day, I was satisfied with my performance. Not that it was good at all — it was horrible. But once I got past my unrealistic goals, I accepted that I had done my best even though my best for that evening was putrid. I was peaceful and comfortable knowing that it was over and there wasn't any reason to look back on it. It was like a revelation that I didn't need to dwell on the evening, that I was only a juggler, just a man and that few things really mattered. The only thing that truly mattered at that time was that I got up. I learned that it took all the talent and skill I had to do the worst performance of my life and then get up and walk away from it. The best juggling, I learned, occurred after the drop.

I didn't always have that knowledge. For most of my life I had created a set of standards, believing there was a right way and a wrong way to live, assuming perfection was possible. Only a few years earlier, I would get terribly angry when I dropped while juggling. I'd throw my clubs, stomp around and curse myself because I wasn't perfect. And I demanded perfection in everything I did. As a high school wrestler, I tore at myself when I didn't win or gave up in despair because I wasn't the best. On the comedy stage, if audiences didn't laugh, I felt I must have done something wrong. Then I got angry and refused to let the anger go. Unfortunately, I applied my standards of living to my family or at least expected them to have high standards of their own. When they didn't, I became even more frustrated. While my demands for perfection and high standards were well-intentioned at first, they grew annoyingly trivial. I was in danger of my world being thrown into disarray by an unexpected TV plot twist. "Oh no. Gilligan broke the professor's radio. Now they'll never get off the island!" I remember arguing with Cheryl once after I had grilled her about how thick she sliced some cheese. I was prepared to defend my views on the thickness of cheese?! Besides being trivial, my standards were unrealistic. Be perfect at juggling? Who could be? What I ultimately learned in St. Louis and during the following year was that there is no such thing as a perfect life. There are as many versions of perfection as there are ways to juggle, many standards to live by and many ways to live. One moment you're striving for perfection, the next moment you're just happy to be alive.

Almost a year after the convention, I suffered an even greater fall. In January of 1992 a slight pain in my knee grew until I could hardly get inside a compact car. I'd had knee surgery from a high school wrestling injury which made the pain seem familiar and non-threatening, and a tumor, much less a cancerous one, was the furthest thing from my mind. The first two doctors I saw confirmed my expectation that I had a simple athletic strain. One said it was a pinched nerve in my back, and the other thought I still had cartilage in my knee from the high school operation. After a magnetic imaging x-ray proved them both wrong, I was told there was a 98% chance that it was only a giant-cell benign tumor.

I should have been leery from the beginning with the two mis-diagnoses, but I hardly gave the latest opinion another thought. But even if I had been leery or questioned the doctors' opinions more, I still could have never expected what lay ahead of me. More so than balls or clubs ever were, even more so than when I messed up in St. Louis, when I finally got the definitive diagnosis of cancer, my entire life was scattered above me in the air. I can't say for sure if I would have felt the same if I hadn't had a change of perspective at the competitions, but in knowing I had cancer, I could apply the knowledge of what I had recently learned — that jugglers drop, that real juggling was dealing with whatever was thrown at me and that, no matter what happened, I could always pick up and start again.

So of all the things I could worry about once I began my one year battle against cancer, my greatest fear wasn't pain, the anguish I knew others would feel or dying at the age of 30. My most pressing concern after diagnosis was whether I would ever juggle again. While, logically, I knew that didn't make sense, it was the first fear to cross my mind. Other fears eventually would follow, but, at the moment, an aggressive tumor was in my body threatening to leave my children fatherless and my parents son-less while, in my head, I was hoping to retain my carnival skills.

I can see it was a form of denial. It reminds me of a night years ago while on the road with a woman I used to work with. While we were driving back from a show in South Dakota, we lost control of our rental car and slid down a six foot embankment into three feet of snow in the middle of nowhere. We were completely stranded at one o'clock in the morning with no one in sight and, while rifling through her things, the first thing she said was, "I can't find my wallet." "Your wallet!?" I said. "We're miles away from anywhere. I think we should be more interested in having our dental records so they can identify our remains." Although her first impulse was irrational, it was genuine, similar to the unusual view I had of my cancer. After all, what good was juggling going to do me it I didn't survive?

It was important because it was my job. I knew it was vital that I support my family: If I died my family would have been better off than if I lived and couldn't juggle. As far as careers go, juggling was the only thing I knew how to do. And aside from being my job, it was simply the thing I knew best. So when everything was about to be taken away, my life itself in danger, I longed to have my career back. I needed to picture myself juggling again. Looking at it that way, my off-beat concern didn't seem so unusual — like a corporate executive's life being completely shaken and his power taken away, thinking affectionately of one day again firing the entire clerical staff. My feelings were like a long since retired baseball player wanting to make a comeback or one of the Wallendas after a fall. Maybe my desire to juggle again wasn't all that irrational. Metaphorically, I wasn't the only one who wanted to juggle again. The corporate exec and the baseball player are jugglers too. The stay-at-home mom, the student, the famous, the obscure — they're all jugglers. As I learned in St. Louis, life *is* juggling. That was what I wanted, to juggle my life again. I wanted the responsibilities of raising my family, finding work and creating new material for my show. I needed to juggle on stage again, to hold some clubs in my hands again, to move my body and strain for a trick. I didn't want to lay around in a hospital bed and depend on chemo or rely on a doctor to run my life.

From diagnosis through all my chemos and operations, when juggling had been taken from me, I was confident that, given another chance, I would be a better juggler than I ever was — on every level. But the diagnosis had been made, the operations had been done and there I was in early May of 1992 in a hospital bed with a Hickman catheter implanted near my heart receiving chemo 24 hours a day. An empty room, a hard hospital bed and a nurse who checked on me hourly — no props, no audience, no responsibilities to make it feel like the balancing act it was. All that was left to juggle were my memories, hospital visits and what lay ahead.

Throughout chemo, as my mind and body were being ravaged, I pictured myself performing again. Even though chemo stripped me of my hair, and operations left me on crutches, I had visions of working at an old comedy club in Minneapolis called J.R.'s that had been closed for years. That showed how far I, subconsciously, wanted to go back in time. Even the club I dreamed of working in didn't exist anymore. But never did my vision feel like a distant or deluded dream. I made plans in my head each weekend after getting out of chemo, feeling certain I would be back on stage. While in chemo, I closed my eyes and I saw myself walking on crutches down to the club, hobbling up on stage with a big smile, telling some jokes about what I was going through and maybe even throwing a few props around. I pictured the crowd loving it. I pictured them, for a minute, living what I was living — laughing about it and being happy. I pictured them forgetting their own troubles by living mine. For the time on stage, they would be a part of my life and I would be a part of theirs. It felt so real. Then I leaned over and threw up into a spit pan, suggesting it wasn't as close as I thought. Sometimes it didn't seem as real as it did at other times. But I kept the vision. And in the meantime, I had my family, friends, a pen to write with, visitors, roommates and the medical staff to help me through the rest.

And though like other patients I had help, I knew cancer was something I had to face on my own. So, having been in comedy for nearly 10 years and juggling for over 15, I looked at my ordeal as another gig. I had done my juggling and comedy show in more clubs than I care to remember. I'd done it for corporate executives, women's groups, high school kids, at countless festivals, in malls, in tents and in the rain. I once got paid to do my show for a man, his wife and their 12-year-old daughter in a hotel room which, taken out of context, I could have been arrested for. I've done national sales meetings, business presentations, store openings. I did a show at a junior college in their cafeteria during lunch and almost none of the students even knew I was there. I performed with Sideshow for over five years. Back when I first started in 1981, I was even doing shows at libraries for pre-school kids and their moms. I had done my show in every place imaginable. Surely I could work a hospital.

Like being booked at a terrible club, I had no option to walk out on my operations and therapies so I made the best of it — letting it be funny, looking for material, or at least something to make me smile. I'm not a look-on-the-bright-side person, but finding comedy in the world of medicine gave me the positive attitude every patient needs. At times it seemed as if my only choices were comedy or paralyzing fear. The two weren't mutually exclusive, and often went hand in hand. Comedy, for me though, was the easiest to recognize.

When I first started visiting the orthopedic surgeon who did all my surgeries, Dr. Roby Thompson, I couldn't help but notice that wherever he went he was followed two or three feet back by med students studying his techniques. They never said or did much of anything. But just being there in their white lab coats and standing in the background trying to fit in gave them an unintentional stooge-ish quality. They were the very definition of lackeys and were fabulously unprepared to interact. When one of the students entered, I said "hi" and he seemed genuinely surprised that I could actually see him. While coughing, he quietly let out a "hi" as his eyes drifted downwards — not unlike the way I responded to girls in junior high.

The students hanging in the background saying nothing reminded me of gangster movies in which a couple of thugs are always at the side of the mob boss. They looked like medical bouncers safeguarding the doctor. I felt as if, should I disagree with the doctor's opinion or dispute a treatment, the young assistant would lean forward, touch the doctor's shoulder and whisper in his ear, "You want I should rough him up for you boss?" It was only a matter of time, I figured, before insurance companies used the students in that capacity. The costs they'd save on reduced second opinions alone would get them to at least think about medical enforcers.

Using humor took the edge off of the paralyzing fear. It was already intimidating being in a sterile room surrounded by three physicians with my pants around my ankles while sitting on that hard white paper butchers use for wrapping meat. Every time I found myself in that position my mind wandered, pretending we were all in some weird comedy sketch. Using humor helped prepare me to hear anything Dr. Thompson could have told me.

"Mr. Burton, the test results are back and I'm sorry to say you have ... gum disease."

"I'm afraid it's bad news. It looks as if you have a terrible case of ... tennis elbow."

"We think, Mr. Burton, you are suffering from worms. We're very sorry."

Any of those diagnoses would have been inconvenient and had me shopping in a different section of my pharmacy, but if I had a choice, I would have happily chosen either of those instead of cancer. Given the option I wouldn't have minded if Dr. Thompson had said, "It seems, Scott, that you have a serious case of PMS." At least that could have explained a few things about my personal life.

Those jokes I played in my head ultimately helped me for when reality finally came around. Because when Dr. Thompson, a sensible, down to business guy, gave us the final diagnosis, the first thing I did was make a joke. It wasn't even a conscious thing. After Dr. Thompson came into the examining room with two med students on his heels (Curly and Moe, I believe) and told us I had cancer, I instinctively quipped back. Actually he never said the word cancer. What he said was, "We've got the reply from Sloan Kettering, and we're pretty sure it's a high grade sarcoma."

"What about the Mayo Clinic?" I responded. "Didn't you send them a sample of the biopsy too?"

"He doesn't have a final opinion. He wants to keep it and re-test it."

I turned to Cheryl and said, as if confidentially, "That way he gets to keep charging, run up a tab and make more money." The joke was that a reputable Mayo clinic doctor would actually try to pad a diagnosis. Admittedly, it wasn't a great joke. But Dr.

Thompson paused a moment and, with the slightest hint of a laugh, said, "You're going to need that sense of humor in the coming months." I thought to myself, "Well, I sure h*ope* I'll need humor. Without juggling that's the only thing I've got left."

But even if I hadn't made a joke, I still wouldn't have had much of an outward response. Like not knowing I was nervous in St. Louis and shying away from social situations, I internalized the diagnosis. Fear was still present. But I wasn't one to grab my doctor by the lapels and say, "I can't have cancer! Why, I've never even been to Europe. There's so much I need to do, I'm not done yet. I need to tell my wife I love her. I ... I want a red sports car. What about skydiving? I've never done that. Madonna hasn't written back to me yet." But melodrama wasn't my style. When faced with cancer I didn't see my life flash before my eyes, it dawdled. I didn't know exactly what having cancer meant, but I assumed I'd have time to figure it out. Before I could consider staging a melodramatic scene, I had a lot of living to do, and laughter and love were at the top of my list.

A Fear By Any Other Name

When I made the joke to Cheryl about the Mayo doctor trying to squeeze money out of us, Dr. Thompson, before he smiled, gave me that same look a mother gives her son when he's noisy in church. It was a momentary stare as if I'd just done something socially out-of-sync. His head shook just slightly in resignation or disbelief as a faint smile eventually crossed his face. I had tried to get Dr. Thompson to break his composure since our first visit to his office. Everyone at the hospital knew him as one of those rare people that emanated respect — a no-nonsense, unflappable, grounded and yet personable human. His presence was so commanding it gave me the uneasy feeling that, even though I knew he was my doctor and all, he could have me fired. And I was self employed! So, being a comic, I cracked jokes to break up any tension that existed — a little for myself, a little for him and a little for the other staff in the clinic. Until that day, Dr. Thompson hadn't laughed at even one of my jokes. It's funny that the one day he finally did laugh was the day he told me I had cancer. But, knowing he had spent years having to tell patients terrible things they didn't expect, I enjoyed giving something to him *he* didn't expect. My one joke bridged two worlds and I liked making that connection.

Everytime I laughed about what I was going through, I felt like another connection was made, either with Cheryl or the medical staff or whoever was in on the laugh. Many times the connections were made only with myself, a little laugh to keep my eyes open and pay attention to the struggle going on around me. I needed those connections to make it through. I needed more than just knowing I had cancer and gee, wasn't that just terrible.

When I went to the University of Minnesota hospital for my biopsy I had an upbeat attitude, I thought. Yet it was as if there were messages all around me telling me how much there was to be afraid of — tears in my mother's eyes, blank stares from my comic friends, do's and don'ts from a dietician. And, not unlike when I bought a new car and all of a sudden I noticed how many other cars exactly like it were on the road, when I was going into the hospital I seemed to hear more horror stories about hospital stays. I didn't want to hear them. But either a friend would tell me so I would be aware or I'd read something in the paper or I'd be in line at Cub Foods and overhear the fellow in front of me tell the story of a friend of some guy's brother who had an uncle that went into a hospital to have his appendix taken out and accidentally had his foot removed and re-attached to his shoulder. With all the messages — talking to friends, medical staff and even my family — I gathered that I was supposed to not only be afraid of cancer, but of the hospital, of my surgery, of rehabilitation, of my future. Not that fear didn't have a prominent place in my life, but I didn't get it. I loved my life. I loved my family, my job, growing up (even growing up alone), working out, jug-gling. There were few things I didn't love. Yet, when I got cancer, I was supposed to switch gears and start worrying about every-thing I loved and fearing everything else? It didn't make sense. The two had to balance somewhere. So, as I entered the hospital, I remembered all the stories and fearful looks but, I also remained confident. I did, however, entertain ideas of putting "do not open" stickers everywhere on my body except my right leg.

Cheryl brought me in and waited with me until I was brought down to surgery. After getting blood removed and statistics taken in a little room on the seventh floor and putting on some thick leg hose and a not-at-all adequate robe, I was ready for a runner to come up and escort me down to surgery. She was accompanied by a thin, bearded fellow in a white lab coat, armed with a clipboard. I was ready to walk down with him, meeting them at the nurses station, when the man said to me, "You're Scott?"

"Yes, I am," I said.

"You're going to have a little work done on your arm, huh?"

"No. My leg."

"Oh," he said, flipping through the pages on his clipboard. "The left one?"

"Well, no. The right one."

He paused a moment then said, "Okay. Well good luck." He said it with a nonchalant air, almost as if he had only been quizzing me to make sure I was the right person allowed to go down for surgery and not some non-patient who was trying to finagle myself into a free operation. "Okay?" I thought. "Okay?!" How could he have that misinformation and simply say, "Okay, let's go perform some major invasive surgery. I'm sure we'll get it figured out by the time you get downstairs to the operating room."

For a moment, visions ran through my head of a dangerous hospital mistake and a little demon appeared on my shoulder saying, "I told you so. I told you so." But, by the next second, I began laughing to myself. It was funny to me how the guy couldn't have possibly been more wrong unless he had said, "So, you're here to have a baby, huh?" With each mis-spoken statement a smile bigger than the last crossed my face. The laughter offset his error and kept me in balance: The worst was not going to happen because I was paying enough attention, but neither was the operation going to be an ideal perfect thing either. I wasn't going to lose any vital body parts nor was my surgery going to be the equivilant of a back and shoulder rub by Cindy Crawford. My prospects were balanced somewhere in between.

I told myself a variety of things after that guy got my information wrong. Maybe he had the wrong chart. Maybe *he* was trying to make a joke. Maybe he was testing me. Or just maybe every ounce of potential ineptness within the entire hospital had been channeled through that one man and had gotten itself all out. No more mistakes could be made because their quota was filled. "If nothing else," I told myself as the young woman led me down to surgery, "at least I wasn't going with *that* guy."

I was pleased with myself that I wasn't afraid when that happened, but, when I told others the story of that guy's mistake, two separate friends said, "Oh my, that is so scary" which left me a little disappointed because I was thinking of putting the bit in my act. I didn't even bother telling them the rest of the operation procedure for fear of making them feel worse than they did when I told them I had cancer.

Although I had several different operations (and a couple of the same ones) and they all had interesting characteristics of their own, the pre-operation process always ran the same — a little bit scary in itself. The pre-op was the place where, before each surgery, I lay on a gurney with half a dozen other specimens in a large, chilly, sterile room, separated by linen drapes as doctors, nurses, trainees, runners, and assistants shuffled about looking for their respective patients. It felt like a fabulously imperfect science as the staff seemed to wander the room aimlessly, which filled me with no overwhelming feeling of confidence. I knew once I saw Dr. Thompson everything would run as smooth as I could hope. The problem was I never saw him right away when I arrived in the pre-op room. It was filled with medical professionals playing musical patients. For a brief time I would be poked and prodded and, occasionally, correctly identified. It wasn't until each of the staff practiced the knowledge of their respective professions on me that I would finally see Dr. Thompson. I knew then, if nothing else, I was at least going to have the *right* operation.

Until I saw Dr. Thompson, it was all the same. The same cold room. The same impersonal parade of staff. The same gurney ride to the surgery bay. The prep room, out of necessity due to so many gaseous drugs being used, had a ventilation system that exchanged the air every thirty seconds. The result was a constant cold breeze flowing through an indoor room with bright lights. As surreal as a wind blowing through a room with no windows appeared, the staff was armed with a pleasant and comforting remedy — my favorite pre-op perk. There was a large warming oven in which they stored thin wool blankets that were brought to each patient upon request. In an otherwise uncertain, rather compromising situation, those blankets were reassuring delights. What made them extra special was the personnel were there to fetch them for me and wrap them around me. Each time I asked for another I felt like a Roman nobleman at the Forum.

"Uh, yes. You, young person."

"Yes, Mr. Burton."

"I feel a chill. Please bring me something warm."

"Yes, Mr. Burton."

"Oh, and you, please don't go too far. I may need another."

"Okay, Mr. Burton. Anything else?"

"Yes. Bring down the young fellow who gets all the information wrong. He amuses me."

What I didn't remember feeling throughout any the processes, operations and chemo was fear — at least outwardly. The fear *was* there, it just didn't make it to the surface. But fear has always been part of my life.. As far back as I can remember, I was afraid of being alone, afraid of having friends, afraid my family didn't love me, afraid of losing, afraid of being on stage, afraid for the world, afraid for my children, afraid of what was going to happen to me after I died. From my point of view, if looked at properly, there was nothing not to be afraid of.

Eventually all of these fears led me to humor. I remember one day, while lying on my bed as an adolescent, I realized that there was so much I could be afraid about that I couldn't afford to be afraid. If I were to be afraid of everything that was fearful I, literally, wouldn't have time for anything else. There was so much to fear it was, ironically, funny. That became the first profound joke that helped me use humor in expressing fear. And not only fear, but joy, love, my very self. I used it on Dr. Thompson, on my high school wrestling team, while facing cancer, on my wife and kids, on anyone I had contact with. Fear and humor were present in my every relationship, but I didn't realize it until I had cancer. Up until then I just thought it was cool that I didn't seem to feel afraid. I thought laughter was my replacement for fear, not an expression of it.

When the anestheiologist came to my gurney in pre-op to poke a few needles in my arm, I asked him if he didn't have something like one of those nicotene patches instead. When I was being led down to the surgery bay I called out like it was happy hour at a bar, "Catheters for everybody. On me!" If it had been appropriate to juggle something down there I would have. I wasn't desperately vying for attention, but I was easing my fears. I was looking for that balance. As a comic, how could I not want to bring in humor? For the brief moment I encountered either medical staff or fellow patient, I wanted them to laugh, to know my name — to have a human relationship. I've never been good at social situations, small talk or first meetings so all I ever want to make clear is that I'm a human being. When I meet people for the first time, I usually try to make them laugh to show their humanity too. In this instance, I was having cancer for the first time. Using humor in this frightening situation told all of us we could still be human.

Going in for my first surgery was a little bit like meeting someone for the first time. Neither of us knew exactly what to expect from the other and were both trying to set each other at ease. I wanted to make a good first impression as I think they did as well. And, because I hadn't had any bad medical experiences up till then, I was even a little anxious to get to know the hospital, to see inside a big-time medical facility. I was wide-eyed, curious and a little chatty. I was like a young new GI in a battle zone, anticipating seeing professionals at work and what life was like at the front. But if I was a new recruit on my first visit wanting to make a good impression, by the end of my stays I had become a model battle veteran, more captivated with the numbing effects of local anesthesia than the surgeries themselves. After the removal of a pin from my knee (surgery number four, I think) the local left me with no feeling in my right leg, yet the simplest twitch sent my foot kicking out of control like a dis-coordinated field goal kicker. I gathered all the nurses around, "Watch this. Watch this!" I squealed like a child with a new toy. And, when the nurses gathered, I did my little trick and called out excitedly, "I didn't *mean* to do that!" They all stared at me like I just showed them how I could touch my nose with my tongue, barely offered up a condescending, "Wow," then moved on to patients who needed the kind of help they could do something about. The relationship was made. Both the hospital and I were comfortable with each other and, if I had become a battle veteran, perhaps I was more of the corporal Klinger type, bucking hard for a section 8.

The personal relationship between the hospital and me was established the minute I woke from the biopsy surgery. I felt around for all my significant body parts and, with them all being where I last left them, I knew I could trust the hospital. And since I was still on the inside of the building, they trusted me. We kept an eye on each other anyhow, but things were headed in the right direction. The snap judgment of trusting the hospital was made not only due to an even number of limbs on my body but also because of the extreme comfort they gave me. The drugs I was on must have played some part in my comfort but the good feeling seemed mostly the result of an extra foam layer laid between the hospital bed and me. It was a thick, spongey foam with indentations like an egg carton that allowed my body to sink into the bed in pure convalescent bliss. I grew to feel as strongly about that fabric as a man who has found his favorite chair. The combination of the soft cushy mattress along with the warm wool blankets almost made the venture into the hospital worth it. Having the biopsy was doing something unpleasant, which was made up for by the perks — like spending the extra $900 to ride in first class just so I can get my drinks for free. Normally I wouldn't have any affection for the hospital process, but, when it came to the blankets and soft bed, I turned into a child with a favorite teddy. I may as well have been wearing a flannel, footie, zip-up nightie saying, "Looky. I have a blanky."

And I was enjoying the comfort. As far as I was concerned, the tumor was gone, I tasted a new experience and I was going to have a good excuse for lying around the house doing nothing. When Dr. Thompson walked in, sat down and said he was sending samples of my biopsy out for other opinions as to what the tumor was, I had almost no reaction, maybe because I was feeling so good. In my head I thought, "Hmmm, well, if they don't know what it is that must mean it's not cancer. A reputable hospital like this can certainly recognize cancer when they see it." Fear had not made itself present yet, not that I would have recognized it if it had.

I was slow to catch on. What Dr. Thompson meant was he sent the biopsy out because he didn't know what *kind* of cancer it was. The second he said they didn't know what it was, any clear-thinking human would immediately assume, "Oh no, that means it's cancer." Maybe he thought I was being brave instead of ignorant, but I wished I had a better reaction than I did. Maybe I was stunned or confused, still high on drugs or just too darned comfortable to care, but I remember saying to him, with the tone of someone who was reading a book and trying not to be disturbed, "All right." But I *wasn't* reading a book. I wasn't even distracted. I was looking right at the man when he told me I had an undeter-mined fast growing tumor in my leg and all I said was, "All right."

I wasn't trying to be funny. If I was, I would have said, "Sure, but how's the *other* leg?" I hadn't made the connection that it could be cancer. It wasn't a question of using humor or understanding fear because, as far as I was concerned, I didn't have concrete information. I kept the door open though. When he had a more complete diagnosis, I would react more appropriately. Until then I embraced a line from a favorite poem of mine called the "Desiderata": "Nurture strength of spirit to shield you in sudden misfortune." Not only did I nurture my spirit for a shield, not only did I try to keep it all in balance with humor, but I *also* had a warm blanket and a foam bed.

I Dream Of Nurse Jeanie

After the doctors had finally concluded that it was cancer in my thigh bone, the next step was to return me to the hospital and have the tumor removed. I would become familiar with the University of Minnesota hospital as I would be in and out if for nearly the next year. Having had a brief stay due to my knee surgery back in high school, I expected the same amount of recovery time. This week, however, would show me that I was in for something completely different. I had more doctors visiting me, more x-rays taken and a more watchful eye over me. From the moment I woke after surgery, I knew I was in for more than a typical hospital stay.

Unlike the biopsy, this surgery involved Dr. Thompson not only removing the tumor, but, to completely rid myself of cancer, removing the bone as well. The operation was called a cadaverous allograph. More simply put, it was a bone transplant, an amputation and replacement of part of my thigh bone. Dr. Thompson explained that he would go in, disconnect the muscles from my femur, remove the infected piece, then replace it with a bone from a bone bank. The words reverberated in my head, "A bone bank, a *bone* bank." Not only did I never want to make a deposit at a bone bank, I was thanking God that I didn't have to visit a teller. Except for the vision I had in my head of hundreds of bones hanging on strings like sides of beef in a meat locker, the operation didn't sound all that special. Although a bone transplant didn't seem out of the realm of possibility to me, Dr. Thompson said encouragingly that the operation was a ground breaking procedure and that only 15-20 years ago someone with my cancer would have faced an amputation.

I liked that he let me know exactly what was going on and how radical and innovative the surgery was. I felt as if I was tasting the cutting edge of medicine, but, deep down, as long as I was assured the tumor would be removed I didn't care what they had to do. They could have used a mellon baller for all I cared. I didn't need an itemized, detailed list to buy into a life-saving procedure. Dr. Thompson could have told me anything and I would have bought it: "The surgery, Scott, entails our team of doctors opening up your leg, taking out the bone, turning it upside down, putting it back in, flipping you on your stomach, taking the bone out from the other side, putting it back right side up, and then spinning your gurney around. Whoever the table points to gets to sew you back up." And I would have said, "Okay, where do I sign?"

Cheryl was more worried about the operation than I was. As the day got closer, neither of us had discussed our feelings about the allograph. We borrowed a bed from our neighbors and readied a separate room for me so I wouldn't have to climb the stairs on crutches, preparing for, but not talking about, the surgery itself. Because I still considered all my medical experiences as positive, I viewed the allograph as a simple, necessary step to fighting cancer. Cancer was the main issue for Cheryl too, so we had talked about that: How did I get it? How would the kids handle it? And what about my parents and siblings?

Finally, the night before the operation, Cheryl told me how concerned she really was. We were cuddled together on our living room couch with a single light illuminating our house. After several minutes of not talking, just holding, looking around the house and thinking of our future, we looked at each other and Cheryl finally said, "For some reason I'm afraid I'll never see you again." The words caught me off guard. I was hardly thinking of the surgery, much less of anything going wrong. I pulled back to look at her face and, in an instant, what started as a quiet, simple time of thoughtfulness became a highly emotional moment. If Hollywood had its way, the second I looked at Cheryl, stirring violin music would have swelled up in the background. The camera would pan in for a tight close-up, her face would be lit against the darkened room, her eyes shining and passionate. Trembling lips and facial twitches would fill the screen as she fought back tears. Throw in a couple of big name stars and a car chase and the academy would have loved it. But every gimmick a director has ever used to yank our heartstrings paled compared to that moment. She was scared. I held her again saying, "Of course you'll see me."

Nothing more was said. I felt bad knowing I couldn't make her fears go away — that I didn't even know she *was* afraid. After she went to bed, and I was packing for the early morning surgery, her words haunted me. *"I'm afraid I'll never see you again."* Were they prophetic? *Should* I be worried? Was that guy who screwed up my biopsy information doing the surgery? I still couldn't fathom what could possibly go wrong during an operation on my leg that would mean we would never see each other again. I couldn't see the doctor saying, after surgery, "Mrs. Burton, the operation on your husband went very well. The entire tumor was removed and his leg is healing properly. Unfortunately, we seem to have lost the *rest* of him."

My attitude was "Let's wait and see before we worry about this. For all we know the operation could go really smoothly." Waiting before coming to a conclusion of what might happen made sense to me. For instance I also didn't understand what Dr. Thompson meant when he said, after the allograph, I would be left with roughly 80% of the use of my leg. I didn't understand not using 100% of anything. Even in my comedy show I always go full throttle. I don't know how to only give 80%; I always give 100% or, if you believe my old wrestling coach, 110%. What would eventually happen — if Cheryl would see me after the operation or how much of a leg I would be left with — would make itself known in due time.

I had thought Cheryl was irrational before my operation, but sometimes people were fearful for me even after I had already gotten through it all. For example, when I told friends and other cancer survivors that my surgery took over nine hours, they were often taken aback: "Nine hours?!!" they would say, "Wow, that's terrible!" But I heard nine hours and thought, "Yeah, that's about right." In my mind I reasoned, "Well, yeah. You don't just *plunge* into a human body. You take your time, make sure you've done things right. Heck, most of us take the time to shampoo our hair twice! If we can take the time to lather, rinse *and* repeat, why shouldn't the doctor take his own sweet time with delicate surgery. Then he's going to want to take a break, have lunch, maybe call home. You have to account for some slush time in there." It didn't occur to me that the anesthesia had virtually shut my body down and that my system couldn't handle that kind of altered state for long. I neglected the whole anesthesia factor and, absent-mindedly, assumed the nurses had simply lulled me to sleep for the surgery. Not understanding the intensity of the operation was my own brand of irrational thought, but, fortunately, my ignorance served me well at the time.

Because of my willingness to wait until situations made themselves apparent, I grew to develop a perspective that every step in life was a leap into the unknown — the best laid plans of mice and Scott always go astray. My marriage, for example, was a leap. As much as I loved Cheryl, as much as I knew I wanted to spend my life with her, she grew to be a completely different person within five years — and so did I. And everything else in my life has been a leap: school was a leap, having children, even simple conversation. So even if I would have factored in the anesthesia, there was no guarantee my operation would have gone as expected. Heck, Cheryl wasn't even sure I'd *survive* it! I don't know how true to my philosophy I've been for the rest of my life, but I saw each step of our one-and-a-half-year cancer ordeal as one huge leap after another.

A couple of years later I crystallized that thought at a diner while having lunch with my brother-in-law, Michael, who was having marital problems. I shared with him my philosophy that I had held most of my life, that once you can handle the worst in life, the rest can be a breeze. For shock value, I used a disgusting example to get my point across. "Life is," I said, "a huge pile of, for lack of a better word, crap." Michael didn't flinch. He just kept looking at me, no nod of the head, no smile of affirmation. Afraid I was going to lose him, I went on. "Not that it's a bad thing, but in the pile, in a big huge vat that is our life, is all kinds of muck, sewage, compost and garbage. And every new experience is a jump into that vat."

Having known me for almost twenty years, he must have had a hunch that this analogy wouldn't be as negative as it sounded. So he let me continue. "I'm not saying life *is* crap. I'm saying life is hard work — and we never know what is coming next, even the good stuff. So every single step in life puts us in that unexpected

muck and *real* life is in the climbing out of that vat. For you it's
dealing with your family. For me it's cancer, my family, learning to
be a human — everything! It's sitting in that crud with ooze
squishing between my toes and saying, 'Okay, here I am. Now how
do I get out of this?' Sometimes climbing out is hard work, other
times it's easy, but the joy, the purpose in all our lives, is in climbing
out and cleaning ourselves off. We're always told how great life is,
but the greatness is not in what we have or get to do, it's in the
challenge. It's getting in the mix of life and living it, not being afraid
of jumping back into the vat because you're going to be back there
again anyhow. Nothing can keep us down knowing we will be in
the vat as long as we are committed to climbing out."

Michael smiled slightly, nodded and looked suspiciously at his
cheeseburger. Maybe he didn't agree, but I think he understood.
"What separates us as humans," I slogged on, "is, because of the
huge expectations people have in life, some folks just stand there in
the festering pile of goo with their hands raised above their heads
saying, 'Oh my God. Eeeeeyuuu. Blech. Ick ick ick. Ptooey.' Even
when things are going well, they still stand in the muck waiting for
someone to pull them out, preferably Ed McMahon with a 10
million dollar check." Michael and I finished our lunch with him
not saying anything more about it and me thinking I needed to
work on my metaphors.

When my cancer experience began after my biopsy, little did I
know what I was in for. When Dr. Thompson told me they didn't
recognize my tumor, I thought I'd be climbing out of the vat
without even a foul smell on me. Maybe Ed McMahon would even
be there with a small check for all my troubles. I hadn't a clue that,
when I got there, there was a vat-keeper in charge. He was a short,
disease infested guy with warts and moles who looked a little like
Tom Bosley from Happy Days in an elf suit, rubbing his smelly
hands and saying, "You might as well get used to it here pal. You're
going to be here for a looooong time."

Tom Bosley notwithstanding, my cancer story truly began after
the allograph surgery. The operation went as well as it possibly
could. Dr. Thompson removed every bit of the cancer which was
an amazing and thankful feat. I didn't know how successful it had
gone because I was so drugged up when I first awoke. I was in a
small room on a gurney trying hard to remember where I kept my
fingers. After bouts of attempting to wake myself up in the

recovery room, the first thing I remembered was being transferred from the gurney to my comfy hospital bed. Cheryl was standing there in my room along with my oldest sister, Arlene and sister-in-law, Amy. My first spoken words during the bed transfer, which had all the delicacy of a beached whale rescue, were to Cheryl. "I told you you'd see me again," I said. Then, not waiting for a reply, I zonked back out in anesthesia land.

The huge amounts of drugs the hospital had given me kept me comfortable, relaxed and worry-free. All I wanted to do was sleep which, having kids, was something I would take any time it was offered to me. In no time the bed began to feel like an old trusted friend. Once I was aware that everything was running smoothly, I was in a great mood to begin a week-long hospital stay. The nurses, though knowing I was content, said to me, "When the anesthesia wears off, call us and we'll adjust your morphine to accommodate any discomfort."

Lulled into a false sense of security, I replied, "Thanks" but was really thinking, "I don't anticipate feeling any pain, so you ladies just go on about your business and don't worry about me." That was an attitude I learned directly from my father who taught all his children that the cheapest form of pain medication was to not complain about it. And, at the time, I had no reason to complain. The residual anesthesia and morphine left me not quite as high as a kite but as high as a good-sized street light. The bed had grown to feel like I was wearing a large set of Nerf clothing and I was due for a sponge bath. The last thing on my mind was discomfort, which was exactly how Tom the vat keeper planned it.

Because I'd had a drug-induced variation of sleep all day, I didn't feel like sleeping that night. It was one or two in the morning when I started feeling something funny in my leg. Strangely, I couldn't figure out what it was. There I was, lying in bed, hooked up to an IV with an enormous bandage wrapping the length of my leg after a full work day of surgery in which most of my leg muscles were removed and reattached, and I was stumped. "Gee, what could that unnatural throb up and down my leg be? Hmmm, let's see. It's not ticklish. It's not an itch. Gee, what *is* that?" Somewhere, way in the back of my subconscious, there was a polite little wisp of a notion that said, "Um ... uh, excuse me but, hey, this hurts. Why don't you call a nurse?" That thought's efforts to make it to my conscious self could be likened to watching little, well-intentioned

Richard Simmons trying to swim to the top of the Empire State building if it were filled with chocolate pudding.

I explained the sensation to the nurse. "It just feels real thick," I said. "Is there anything wrong here?" At that point my nurse seemed even more confused than I was. She was a short and stout woman, young and with a spirited look in her eyes, which made me hopeful she could help me. But luck was not with me that night.

"Maybe you've been lying here on your back too long, " she replied. "Perhaps if we turn you on your side that will relieve any pressure." Because I knew how my leg felt I had a hard time believing her. If my pain was because I was laying on my back too long, why weren't they turning everyone on their sides. I pictured the head nurse saying over the intercom, "Okay ladies, it's 10:30! Time to tip the patients." Without explaining why, she left. Although I hoped she would forget all about my problem, she didn't. She returned in ten minutes with some hired goons who hefted me up on my side. The moment they did, the formerly meek notion of pain burst through the anesthetic blockade like running back Emmitt Smith through a defensive line of preschoolers, dashing into the end zone of my mind and spiking the ball viciously. "HEY, SCOTT! THIS HURTS!"

After being shown what real pain was and having Tom Bosley's face permanently etched upon my psyche, I re-evaluated my earlier position and decided that the swelling in my leg didn't hurt so much after all. I asked the nurse and her thugs to lay me on my back again. I then suggested that pain medication might be a good idea. To my surprise, she didn't agree with my diagnosis. She was considering other alternatives — like waiting until morning. My confidence, knowledge and instincts were finally intact, so I said, "I *need* more pain medication." After she left to get it, I lay there alone with my pain thinking, "Richard Simmons made it."

Though juggling was my first goal at diagnosis, during that night, I altered my perspective drastically. Standing up was my goal, walking on my leg, living without pain. I still hoped to one day juggle, but, in reference to how I felt, how it seemed my recovery would go, it was like Ray Charles hoping to get his hunting license. Once I fell asleep and that night passed, however, my emotions swung as far back to positive as they had to uncertainty the previous evening. I had finally fallen asleep and, in that time, the anesthesia worked its way out of my system. The increased morphine left me mostly pain free, and the previous night's nurse was nowhere to be seen.

To my delight, a new nurse came sprightly into the room with a friendly, inviting smile. I could tell she was a good nurse, or at least one who wouldn't hurt me. While she fixed up the bed next to me for a new roommate, I told her what happened to me the night before. Laughing sympathetically, she said, "Ah well. We're all doing our best. Maybe it's not always perfect, but we try." Later in the day she gave me a sponge bath. When she held me firmly, I felt a gentleness, as if, had I fallen, she would have caught me.

I used to think good nurses were somewhat distant. I imagined them discussing procedures with the doctors, figuring medications and methodically dressing wounds, but the calming, human presence of this nurse showed me there was a quality of nursing beyond medicine. She had an energy, a sense of being there that could help make the hospital stay a growing experience. I thought of it as Zen nursing. This nurse's centeredness, down-to-earth attitude, and earnest conversation provided the best nursing I could have asked for. Without knowing it or even trying, she helped me out of the vat or, as a Zen master might put it, the hospital stay of 1,000 days begins with the first sponge bath.

The next morning I looked for the down-to-earth nurse who rekindled my spirit but instead found one who was more down-to-business. Although she looked a little like Debra Winger in "Urban Cowboy," I couldn't help but be disappointed. Even though the new nurse was good at her job — and probably could ride a mechanical bull — I was already attached to the one who put me at ease.

Intellectually, I knew that shifts and schedules changed, so I couldn't expect the same nurse. Emotionally, though, I felt a little let down by the system. I longed for just one nurse whom I could latch onto and who would be my camp counselor for the length of my stay. And I didn't want to rely on some suspicious call button either. If I needed my nurse I expected to only have to look to my left. Ideally, I wanted the director of the hospital to walk in with an RN and say, "Scott, this is Donna. She's going to be your nurse for the next 168 hours. And after that she's going to have lunch." Unfortunately the hospital was not designed to revolve specifically around me.

The following days my medical schedule turned into a kind of nurse roulette. After Debra Winger, I was with the curly-haired nurse who liked to chat; then, with a spin of the wheel, I had the short, dark-haired, fast-working, quick-talking nurse. One more spin and I got the male nurse who tried so hard to show he wasn't homophobic that he aggressively touched me in places I'd rather not be touched.

I would have preferred the one-nurse system, but the procession of different nurses and the occasional visits from family, friends and orthopedic wanna-bes was a pleasant distraction. It seemed there was always someone new to share stories with or talk about the medical procedure du jour. "There's always somebody doing something," I told friends who visited. "At seven a.m., a group of med students come into my room, tug on my leg and check my bandages. At eight or so, a nurse comes in to check to see if I need anything. After ten, Dr. Thompson comes in to ask if there are any problems. Then either there's a little lag time or someone visits between noon and four and after that, the night nurse comes in to make sure everything's okay when her shift begins. Man! I'm more scheduled here than I am at home."

The visits from family and friends were especially uplifting. When our next door neighbors visited, they gave me a bright yellow, stuffed dinosaur that made a high-pitched squeal when I squished it. My mom stopped by, Cheryl brought the kids and several family relatives came. I appreciated that people were willing to spend their time with me. Every day people came into my room with a purpose, to feel as if they were contributing, to roll up their sleeves and work for the well being of others. They were in the vat with me. Maybe not with the same sludge on their feet, but all of us, whether cleaning, visiting, doctoring or patienting, were in it together. I liked knowing I was part of that group.

On Thursday I got a surprise visit from Debby, who had come all the way up from Omaha. Her visit also helped change my outlook for the rest of my stay. Debby and I have always been able to speak the same language. I told her about when my anaesthesia wore off, about the lack of nurse consistency and how I was due for 12 rounds of chemotherapy, two separate protocols. "Yet," I said to her, "as long as I don't die, it's not that bad of a deal." When I said things like that, I felt some people were skeptical, others patronized me or didn't believe me at all. But Debby understood.

Except for going down for x-rays, Debby was the first person to get me out of my bed by suggesting I take a wheelchair ride. Based on the few bed-to-gurney transfers I'd had, which felt like they were done by disgruntled teamsters, I was leery of moving at all. But we asked the nurse and she thought it was a good idea. Yet I thought it was best not to move from my bed until Dr. Thompson walked in and said, "Well, you're healed. You can go home now." The move to the wheelchair was easy and painless, but in my head I was saying, "I shouldn't be doing this. I shouldn't be doing this. What's going to happen?" It was like I invoked the spirit of Eeyore from the Winnie the Pooh stories, whining in a low moan, "Oh dear. We'll probably end up lost or crashed." My rational mind prevailed and Debby wheeled me down the hall.

After a few days of confinement, that wheelchair ride felt like a European vacation. Moving so quickly, I felt an emancipation, a rebirth into a new world of recovery. She took me outside, and I was giddy with excitement wanting to say to people we passed, "Look at me. Look at me move. Don't I go fast?" My childish excitement, though, was surpassed by the simple and humbling view I had of Debby and me strolling through the hospital commons. It was almost a vision, a God's eye view of us, a young woman pushing a young, debilitated man across a tiny arc of the earth under a sunny, crisp blue sky.

Juggling was still a fun thought and performing a tangible goal, but when I saw our lives as little more than a humble walk on a tiny part of our planet in an enormous solar system, many goals got set on the back burner. Unfortunately, I only could be reverent for so long. On our way back to the hospital, I pointed to a guy across the grassy park area and said, "See that guy wearing the mask? He's on my floor. You know that mask isn't to protect him from germs or anything. It's a feedbag."

The wheelchair ride was empowering. It was a simple matter, but I felt like I was doing something about my own recovery. Another empowering moment was getting up and using the bathroom by myself for the first time ("I'm a *big* boy now!"). I have no specific details about it, but it matched the wheelchair ride in its sense of freedom and in the accomplishment of getting up and walking on my own. Up to that point I had been assisted by a catheter which, going into my operation, was the only thing I knew I didn't want to have. I prayed that I wouldn't have one. I can't imagine anyone not. I prayed so hard against it, it never dawned on me that perhaps I had one anyhow. But midday after the surgery, I wondered out loud to my nurse saying, "With all I've been drinking through last night and today, I wonder why I haven't had to use the bathroom." She replied, and I paraphrase with great license here, "Because we've got you on a leash."

The shock of having a catheter, I'm ashamed to say, was greater than when I was first told I had cancer. It was like I went through the five emotional stages of facing death: denial, anger, fear, bargaining, and finally, acceptance. Lifting my covers slowly as if I had just been told I was a double amputee, I saw that she was right. A huge tube was exiting my body in a place where I never wanted a tube *in* my body. I couldn't fathom how they got it in to begin with. As eager as I was to have it removed, I also was adamant, since it was in already, that nobody touch it. It was a distasteful appendage and hideous to look at, but I had to admit it served its purpose well. I just sat there unable to get out of my head the vision of a camel through the eye of a needle.

It was a rollercoaster week, an appropriate start to a wild, up and down cancer journey. In the movie "The World According To Garp," Garp says excitedly, as if it were a revelation, "It's funny how sometimes you can live a whole life in one day." Then he pauses and adds, "I had a great life today." Each day in the hospital was an incredible life. My body experienced everything from the poking and prodding of the medical staff to the comfort and warmth of family. Each day was an incredible life, the week was an incredible life, my *life* was an incredible life.

The signature moment of my entire hospital stay was a drug-induced dream at the end of the week. Every day I was given four shots in my leg of a drug called Tordol, a muscle relaxant. One night, before my last shot, I was given a sleeping pill as well. It didn't kick in right away, but when it finally did I felt incapacitated, at the very edge of sleep. And that was when the nurse came in with Tordol. I was so groggy that I was aware of her presence, but I couldn't even find the strength to acknowledge her. She gave me the shot and, after pulling out the needle, left the injection site with a small amount of blood rolling away from the skin. It was only a drop or two but I could feel it. It was like the feeling of having a runny nose dripping down my lip, yet I was so drugged that I couldn't even move my hand up from my side to wipe away the blood. It was like I was Batman, after the Riddler had left me in some compromising near death scenario. "If I ... can ... just ... reach ... my ... utility belt ..." Then I fell into the dream.

Strangely, it didn't feel like a dream because, although I was quite sedated, I felt I knew what was going on. In what seemed to be a cross between a doctor's waiting room and a roadside diner, I was sitting contendedly on a Naugahyde couch with a chrome metal frame, listening to muzak. I was really enjoying the tunes, so it *must* have been a dream. Then, one by one, disembodied floating faces of older women entered the room, billowing like cigarette smoke from a blackened room behind me. Each of them held presence just behind me, their faces mutating to the properties of lingering smoke. With each new presence, though not feeling threatened, I flailed at them. I tried to push them back or put their smokey heads in a headlock. When I ignored them, they taunted me further, lingering and hovering. I felt I had to keep sitting there, but the heads kept coming.

The interpretation of the dream hit me one day almost a year later. The fact that I didn't get up from the couch meant I felt I was stuck in the hospital. The changing faces represented the nursing staff. And my reaction of fighting the floating heads was how I adapted to each new nurse. I felt frustrated on every level. While still dreaming, I remember thinking, "Man, if this wasn't a dream, this would *really* be weird." But that was only the beginning, a warm-up to the strange reality I would experience after several months of chemotherapy.

Holy catheters, Batman!

First Week In Chemo

If to the general public cancer is the C-word, then to cancer patients the other C-word is chemotherapy. It is a relatively experimental treatment, originating only 30 or so years ago, and though widely used, is prescribed out of desperation. It wasn't until after my treatment had started that I asked my nurse what exactly chemo was. She told me chemo's job was to kill all the fast growing cells in the body. That included killing the cells lining of the stomach, which caused nausea, the cells in the throat, which produced severe pain, as well as the hair follicles, which could cause baldness. It is, in a word, poison. Chemo's job is to destroy everything in the body, including the cancer. The body is brought to the brink of death in hopes that the cancer is killed before the patient is. I would use the analogy of setting an over-grown forest in flames so that new growth can begin. They are both risky solutions to desperate problems.

Before I knew what chemotherapy was, I had planned a regimen that I was going to follow. The bone transplant robbed me of mobility, which meant I wouldn't be able to jog, jump rope, juggle or maintain any kind of aerobic workout throughout chemo. Determined not to let the fatigue and nausea associated with chemo take away the rest of my body, I planned on doing push-ups and isometrics every day and, as my leg got better, sit-ups. These exercises, I expected, would keep me fit throughout the ordeal and possibly even make me more resistant to pain. I would keep my mind sharp by writing daily, and my spirit buoyant by listening to the music of Van Morrison, Bob Dylan and others who had a profound effect on my soul. Without having set one foot on the cancer clinic floor or knowing what chemo would be like, I'd devised a plan for handling it. That was like the Wright brothers, without ever having flown so much as a kite, charting a journey to the moon.

During the week before I first visited the cancer clinic, my imagination ran wild with what chemo would be like. Would it be hours upon hours of wretched pain? Would I find myself in cold sweats like a drug addict going cold turkey? Like a Vietnam vet or a chemically imbalanced person, would the suffering bring on a dementia that would change how I looked at life forever? I pictured all of those, plus throwing up hourly, plus constant supervision, plus being able to physically see the battle between my cancer and the chemo drugs. My plan to maintain body, mind and spirit was created with those fears specifically in mind.

My first visit to the oncologist, the technical name for a cancer doctor, eased my mind a little. I was relieved that he didn't hook me up to a couple bottles of chemo right away. The week of obsessing and worrying made me want to, at the same time, get it over with and never begin at all. Because I didn't think of chemo to be medicine as much as a last ditch resort, I didn't expect it to require prep time. I thought taking chemo would be like an age-old social ritual. The doctor, I imagined, kept a dose or two of the poison handy — the way my parents used to keep liquor in a high cupboard — with a black skull and crossbones on it. He'd offer me a dose the way one offers a drink and stand by as I hunched over, vomiting after having a little too much. And then he'd offer me more. I knew it would be a sterile, hospital version of drinking oneself sick, with an IV and a comfortable chair and a nurse standing by, but it didn't matter.

After thinking of it in these terms, I was so psyched for getting chemo on the spot, they could have hooked me up in the parking lot and I wouldn't have been surprised. But after checking me out, the doctor said I wouldn't receive a typical four hour out-patient treatment. Instead, I'd have a tube put in my chest and be on a 24-hour-a-day drip in the hospital beginning the following week. Not knowing what getting in-patient treatments meant, I felt lucky —

like I was getting special attention. And after seeing the other folks sitting in vinyl chairs with needles in their arms, not looking like receiving chemo was a social event at all, I was praying that I wouldn't be one of them. So when the doctor told me I would be staying in the hospital, my overall reaction, being shortsighted and thankful was, "Cool."

At the time, I didn't know that receiving chemo as an in-patient meant that my cancer warranted an extra aggressive approach. I just figured the doctor could administer chemo any way he wanted, either in the hospital or in the clinic, and that he chose the hospital just like he arbitrarily chose an external Hickman catheter over an implanted Porta-cath. There were plusses and minuses to each kind of treatment. In the clinic I would be in and out within the day, but I might be leery as to whether I was getting everything I needed. In the hospital I'd have constant supervision, so if anything went wrong, an entire staff was there to take care of me.

The downside was being in a hospital. I wouldn't be home for a week at a time. I wouldn't be in my own element or feel completely comfortable. In the hospital I knew I was getting the most aggressive treatment to fight my cancer, but intense treatment opened the door to the kind of suffering I was trying to avoid. The bottom line was, with either treatment, I would still be getting chemo. And, deep down, that was what I wanted to avoid.

The next Thursday, Cheryl and I walked along the University of Minnesota campus to the Masonic Cancer Center. Both of us felt that what we were experiencing wasn't reality. I was on crutches which made walking side by side difficult. With every step, I was thinking, "Look at this. It's happening. We're getting closer and I'm going to have chemo. We've talked about it, planned for it, even laughed about it, but it's *really* happening. There's no getting out of it." We headed up the sidewalk toward the large sign that stated the building's intentions clearly — Masonic Cancer Center. Next to the sign there were about six people smoking. "Daredevils?" I wondered. Smoking next to a cancer hospital made as much sense as skydiving with a lead-lined parachute. These people reminded me of little kids when their mother has just said, "Honey, don't touch the iron. It's very hot. It will burn you and you'll cry." The child says, "Okay," but then touches the iron, burns himself and cries.

The dream-like feel continued as we reached the third floor,

Masonic 3. We met the nurses at the registration desk and, with every word I spoke, there was a distant feel to it like I was watching it all on TV. "Hi, I'm Scott Burton," I said. "I'll bet you're expecting me." The first nurse said, "We sure are. Why don't I take you down to your room while they finish your paperwork here?"

Her words were so common, so real, which emphasized that no matter how odd being on the cancer floor felt, it sure wasn't television. If it were television, the air would have been filled with urgency, life and death calls pouring into the nurses station, doctors visibly wrestling with experimental treatments and emergency teams speeding down the hall in a flurry of stethoscopes and gurneys. I'd seen "Emergency" and "Rescue 911." I'd seen Chad Everett furrow his brow on "Medical Center." Television is a cheap, scripted version of reality. With nothing to greet me but a sedate nurses station and staff quietly doing there paperwork and tending to patients' needs, I faced reality and abandoned any hope of waking up or changing the channel.

Cheryl and I said good-bye because she had to be with the kids and we both figured the first day would be filled with all sorts of hospital protocol to keep me busy anyhow. She walked toward the elevator as the nurse escorted me to my room. As she led me down the sterile, barren white corridor, I couldn't help but notice how unadorned the floor was. The sparse halls fit in with my image of getting chemo from my doctor being like getting drunk in a back alley, but I was still surprised. In a place where people were desperately ill, some terminal, and many suffering from varying bouts of depression, I thought there should be a sense of decor, color, or something to distract the eyes and spirit. Instead, Masonic 3 had the charm of Jack Nicholson's ward in "One Flew Over The Cuckoo's Nest."

Back at the oncology clinic where children were treated, their unit was decorated like an amusement park, beautiful blue-green walls with dark waves and huge colorful fish painted on them. There were even some large wooden fish sticking perpendicularly out of the walls with their big fish lips poised in a perpetual whistle. *That* , I thought, was how to care for an unsure patient. Compared to the children's clinic, walking onto Masonic 3 was like stepping into the Gulag with nurses. I went from Disneyworld to Dresden all in the same medical facility. Quietly, I grumbled to myself, "I want some fish, darn it. I want some big, colorful, puffy-lipped fish right now!"

What served as my best distraction was the nurse walking me down the hall. She was upbeat, pleasantly cheery and chatty, helping to erase some of my immediate anxieties. I found it hard to believe the nurses on a cancer floor would enjoy their jobs or be pleasant to talk to at all. My vision was that oncology nurses, because they were around cancer all the time, would be dour, straight-faced and sobering. If they went out for a drink after work, I couldn't see them *not* complaining. One nurse would say, "What a day. It's like every one of my patients had cancer." Her co-worker replies, "Well you *do* work in a cancer hospital." "Oh, that's right," the first one recalls. "Man! I hate my job."

The woman who brought me to my room made it appear that oncology nurses were even more positive and engaging than other fields. She was surely a good nurse. I could see in her eyes and hear in her voice that she loved her job. When we reached my bed and I began sorting out my things, that sweet little nurse, bless her soul, chatted about her stories in chemo as she prepared the room. She explained how, as time wore on, she would collect increasingly more hair from each of her patients' pillows every morning. Then, just as I was about to ask why she was collecting the hair at all, she switched to curious stories of her battles with physicians that practiced poor bedside manner and of some patients' problems with not having a living will. While listening I thought little of my own predicament and was intrigued by her commitment to such a difficult job.

With such a talkative nurse, my first moment on Masonic 3 was less like television than radio — which was just what I needed. As it turned out, that nurse was an angel who came during my special need. She made my time informal and natural, even as I was about to go through some of the most *un*natural treatment known to man. With all her peculiarities, she was the perfect nurse to prepare me for and see me through chemo. I'd found the perfect match. I adopted that nurse as my talisman for my cancer journey, my lucky charm. I quickly felt comfortable and at ease and trusted that her smile and talkative manner would help me through the next seven months. Unfortunately, after 5 p.m., I never saw that woman again.

The game of nurse roulette had started all over again. I didn't know it at the time, but through some shift in the nurses' schedules, I was done with the nurse who made me feel so secure. (On the other hand, maybe she wasn't a nurse. Perhaps the gathering of hair was for some massive arts & crafts project that's better left unsaid.) Fortunately I found that all the nurses I had on Masonic 3 were blessed with a similar love of their jobs and patients. I wouldn't have to relive the dread of the post-operative orthopedic floor.

Once I was feeling comfortable and the nurse left to do her other work, a young fellow came in to weigh me and take my temperature. After he was done, I waited for the next person to come in — someone to hook up my chemo, draw blood, give me pills or something. But nobody came. I wanted to get up and leave but thought it would be rude, since the hospital had gone out of its way to make me some extra special chemo and I wasn't even there to receive it. After an hour I went out to the nurses station. "Not that I want to rush you or anything," I said, "but am I supposed to be getting chemo today or is this all just a dress rehearsal kind of thing?"

"No. It's not a rehearsal," the nurse answered. "Your chemo should be here ... What time did you get in today, nine? You should have your chemo by about five or so."

"Five!?" I screamed so loudly in my head I almost had to tell myself to quiet down. "Why on earth would it take until five?" I then asked the nurses, more politely than I asked myself, what caused the delay. They told me that it took especially long to write up the orders and mix the chemicals downstairs. I believed their answer for the first and second weeks, reasoning that maybe there were forms to fill out. Maybe they were making chemo from scratch with nothing but some base elements and a chart of the periodic table. Maybe there was a long line of people waiting with other chemical orders to fill like a really busy day at the deli. If that was the case, I could wait.

That reasoning served me well the first week, but the delay also occurred every following week so that it got to be a kind of joke. Every week I complained and every week they told me that the chemo was still being mixed. Eventually I said, "You'd think that by the fourth or fifth week the people writing the orders might have caught on that I was a regular and send a message first thing saying, 'Hey, Scott's coming again.' Or maybe those people downstairs could make just a little extra next time and keep it in the fridge so that, just once, the treatment would be ready at the same time I was." The nurse would smile kindly and say, "We'll pass the message along."

For this first week, I didn't mind the wait and took the extra time as an opportunity to get familiar with my surroundings. I wanted to get out anyhow because in the short time I sat alone in my room I had begun to worry about things like, "How much pain will I go through" and "What if even after chemo I die anyhow?" Fortunately, because there were no answers to them, these worrisome questions lasted only about twenty minutes before they gave way to less burdensome observations such as, "How come my second toe is longer than my first?" and "I wonder how much my head weighs?"

It was too much time in a place where I really didn't want to be. I could have handled it better if there would have been distractions like the ones at the children's clinic. I could have spent my down time doing spin art or something — playing Nintendo or throwing softballs at an oncologist in a dunk tank. I had my notebook to write jokes and observations in and the nurses let me use a tape player, but I wasn't ready to fall back on those. After all, I hadn't even gotten chemo yet.

Instead of waiting around, I walked the halls. With my physical regimen in mind, I went looking for the workout room — a little weight room or a gym where I could go to keep active. When I was at the nurses station asking about my chemo, a couple of elderly gentlemen were pacing the halls with their IV stands. They, too, weren't going to stay holed up in their rooms figuring out new ways to fold their electric beds. They were fighting back. I was impressed that they made good use of the desolate hall, but being used to a heavier workout, I wanted an exercise room. After one trip up and down the hall, looking in every room and doorway, I realized that those fellows walked the cold tiles between the stark white walls because that *was* their gym. The unadorned hallway with nurses and lunch carts was their gym and they paced it as if doing laps. It was the original Club Med.

I couldn't bring myself to walk the halls: It would have felt like some sort of exercise for the tired prisoners in the movie "Papillion." Knowing that I wasn't going to find a workout space, I wandered to the end of the hall. There I found a small waiting room with a TV, coffee table with magazines on it, and a hard vinyl couch that was the kind of yellow/brown color only hospitals find pleasing to the eye. There was nothing comforting about it and it certainly wasn't an exercise room, but I adopted it as my place, my refuge to write, watch TV or even fashion a workout. I got down, gimp leg and all, and did 50 push-ups. I didn't know it at the time, but that would be my only visit to that room.

Adjusting my views on working out, I reluctantly returned to my own room. After spending several more hours wondering what chemo would be like, turning on and off the TV, checking with my nurses, and staring at the blank pages of my notebook, a nurse came in with an IV and hooked up some fluids and anti-nausea medicine into the Hickman catheter in my chest. Shortly after that, I had my first visitor. Mike, a friend of the family, showed up which both surprised me and made me feel a little guilty. He came to lift my spirits on my first day of chemo and I hadn't even received any yet. I had only wandered around, used the facilities, and played around with some of the floor's equipment. Except for the fluids they'd given me, up to that point I was only on a field trip.

The nurse returned pushing another IV stand with a maze of tubes and switches running up into four plastic bags filled with liquids. Although it looked like a new puzzle from the makers of Rubik's Cube, I knew exactly what it was, and so did Mike. But neither of us acknowledged the severity of what I was about to go through. Because we both knew how bad chemo could be, we kept our emotions in check, and talked as casually as if we were discussing the local baseball team. I said to him, "I've been wondering all day what this is going to be like." As calmly as if he were tossing out pitching stats, he replied, "Yeah, you read a lot of stories of how bad chemo is, but I'll bet you never know how you're going to feel until you actually get it."

Mike was a guy who could talk about anything — music, pop culture, sports or politics — and sound well informed. He'd been studying to be a sign language interpreter and we discussed everything from his classes to Bob Dylan concerts. But he was preoccupied with the terrible smell in my room due to a combination of the medicine smells in the hall and my roommate being a little gaseous that day. Mike was getting so bothered by the smell, I was afraid he was going to get up, poke my roommate in the shoulder and tell him to quit it.

As Mike made another sour face toward my roommate's curtain, I brought the conversation back to chemo. "I see it working like a medical version of that game Mousetrap," I said. "Once the chemo's turned on, it's going to run down from the IV sack, race through the tubes like a lit dynamite fuse, bend and twist all around, reach the catheter connected to my sub-vena cava and, once the poison reaches my heart, I'll shoot a great heave of bile out of my mouth into the metal pan they gave me for catching the stuff."

Mike shrugged with a "who knows?" look on his face because he was in no position to say, "Bet it doesn't" or "That's the stupidest thing I've ever heard." Then we both watched as the nurse flipped the valve letting the chemo run free like a plumber turning on your water. The chemo did twist and bend around the tubes bound straight for my heart, but when it reached me, I felt no different. No sickness, no cold feeling in my chest like I'd just been injected — nothing. "It was the push-ups," I thought. "Not just the push-ups but a life of exercise, wrestling, running, lifting weights, basketball and playing tennis with Jack. All the working out and nurturing my strength of spirit had prepared me." Chemo wasn't going to be as bad as I had imagined.

When Mike left I was upbeat, thinking that fighting cancer was only a matter of spending time in the hospital, not an internal mental, physical and spiritual struggle. Because I was so content, I hadn't even noticed that I hadn't eaten a thing all day even though the nurses encouraged me every hour or so to get some nutrition in my body. As naive as I had been after the bone transplant, I assured them that I would do what I could, but that I honestly didn't see any problem with not eating.

I got my first glimpse of what chemo had in store for me when at the end of the evening I vomited for the first time. It was during a visit from my first and only girlfriend before I got married. I met Linda Harris in 1981 while working at a Renaissance Festival in Kansas City, and as surprising as it was for Mike to be my first visitor, to see her enter my room felt like a remake of "This Is Your Life" with Rod Serling as host.

Linda and I had dated long distance for several years. I was 20, she was 16 and our split was messy and painful, what with me being socially inexperienced and her barely a high schooler. She arrived with a good friend and performing partner, Phil Lindsay, but he left us alone to talk. Linda and I had talked about our uncomfortable parting and battling issues a year or so beforehand, so we met as good friends who had parted ways, lived different lives and were trying to catch up again.

"I can't believe how good you look," she said more than once, indicating she expected to see me looking like the possessed child in "The Exorcist."

"So far it's not so bad," I told her. "I don't have much to go on since it's just my first day, but I really feel fine." We talked about her boyfriend and their trip to Central America by car and how much she liked Dennis Miller's talk show. Looking into her young, pretty face and seeing all the past years while feeling the present at the same time made for one of my fondest visits in the hospital. Each second was like living a lifetime.

And that was the moment my body chose to throw up.

A young girl from Kansas City takes time out to visit an old boyfriend she had no reason to talk to and then that old boyfriend, in the middle of pleasant conversation, woofs a piece of food into a spit tray. Linda was very good about it, perhaps expecting much worse. "Oh, that's okay," she said, trying to downplay it as if this happened whenever she visited old boyfriends. I'm sure she was already concerned about how I was handling cancer, so not only did she not make a big deal of my regurgitating, she seemed a little embarrassed for me. If she could have, to help me be less self conscious, I'm sure she would have put it back for me. She was acting just that sweet.

My disappointment was that I wouldn't have thrown up at all if it weren't for the peach I'd eaten about an hour before. The nurses had been bugging me so much to eat that they had brought me fruit from the kitchen because I said I could possibly eat some. But I didn't feel like eating. I didn't know it because it was so subtle, but it was the effects of nausea. Then, an hour before Linda came, just as quickly as a sick bug can hit a healthy person, out of nowhere, I suddenly felt well. Seizing the opportunity I reached into the bowl, ate a piece of fruit, then proudly called my nurse to tell her I ate a whole peach. Somewhere back at the station I'm sure the woman wanted to say patronizingly, "Oooh, good, Scott. Now lay out your mat for nap time." Then, like a perverted magic act, I made the entire peach reappear in front of a friend I hadn't seen for years.

Once again I was encouraged because, although it was my first time regurgitating, it wasn't *that* bad. It wasn't a curse or horribly painful. It didn't taste bad at all — just a brief spit and it was over. Actually my first reaction was that it tasted rather … peachy.

The Unusual Suspects And
Why I Didn't Think About Death

People sound surprised when I tell them that I didn't think much about death during that time, but it doesn't seem strange to me. At least not any stranger than my life up to that point. There is no doubt that I had an unusual childhood. My parents, who raised six kids in a small south Minneapolis home, were both deaf since infancy. Although their deafness most certainly played a part in how I have come to view the world, as far as I was concerned having deaf parents was no more strange than having an outside relative live with the family.

Because Mom and Dad straddled the hearing and deaf worlds, we kids grew up partially in the deaf community. I remember us kids running up the three flights of stairs at St. Paul's Thompson Memorial Hall, what we and the deaf community called The Clubhouse. We'd run to the other side of the building then down the back staircase, tearing through that place with reckless abandon because we knew we weren't making too much noise for the twenty deaf adults meeting in the basement. We were used to the precise movements of their fingers and the passionate gestures of communicating in sign language; to the loud noises — sometimes grunts, sometimes high-pitched moans — that they made when they were stressing a point; and to their having to talk or finger spell very slowly because we Burton kids had never learned sign language. I remember the Clubhouse and all the deaf people we grew up with fondly and never knew it was different than growing up in a hearing family.

That silence may, in fact, have been why I felt so comfortable with my own as I grew up. I compensated for the outward silence by keeping endless conversations going on in my head. From the earliest moment that I can remember — from playing with my Mattel figurines downstairs in the laundry tub to sneaking between the garages in back as if I were on a special covert mission — I talked to myself in my mind. Those conversations started as benign patter that most kids would say out loud while playing. "Ha ha, I've caught you, Burton," the first voice in my head would say in my hero/spy game. "No you haven't," the second would reply, while I climbed up on the garage, "because I have the power to jump as high as I want." They've stayed with me, not just while playing, but while discussing the current issues of my life. Once, when I had the prospect of becoming better friends with the kids on my park board football team, I was in a quandary as to whether or not I should accept their invitation to go out and do some minor vandalism on Halloween. The thought of doing so made me feel awful so I debated the issue with myself:

"They actually want me to be friends with them," I thought. "It probably wouldn't be so bad."

"Of course it would be awful. They want to throw eggs at houses and steal candy — do *you* want to do that?"

"Well, no. But it's just one night and then I'll get to hang out with them for a long time. I'll bet Jack has egged a few houses."

"But how can it matter whether it's just one night or who else has done it if it's still wrong?"

Fortunately, I had my sister Debby to help me make the decision. She was just about the only person I could talk to about such problems at the time because she was willing to be understanding to me. Even knowing how badly I wanted to have friends, Debby bluntly said to me, "Why do you want to hang around them, Scott? They're jerks."

Because of how easy it is to make friends as I child, without even knowing how, I had a few friends in the neighborhood and some at school even when I wasn't confident in my communication skills. Having practiced all those conversations in my head, with friends to talk to, I not only talked but almost couldn't stop. In some instances I was close to being a loudmouth. I enjoyed a few years of expressing myself until moving on to junior high school. By that time, after my childhood pals expanded their horizons and found new relationships, I felt strange deeming one person a friend and another not a friend and consequently ended up without any.

Not being unfamiliar with it, I went back to being silent. While I certainly didn't want to be lonely, I was comfortable with it. I spent close to five years feeling mostly alone — though finding occasional moments or certain classes at school where I could be my talkative self as well. Having accepted myself as my own best friend because their weren't too many others to choose from, I was the one I talked to about where my life was headed, why I had it and where it was going. Not thinking much of it, I came to a point where I realized that I was living, at separate times, in completely different worlds. I had lived with six kids and deaf parents and was happy. I had friends to play baseball in the street or other games with till dusk with and I was happy with that. And I had my own world where all I had was me and occasionally a bag full of army men, and I was happy with that too.

By the time I was spending most of my time alone — through junior high and most of high school — I started to look for a common thread to connect my wildly different worlds. Maybe I'm just not good at finding the intricacies of possible connections, but the only common bond among my worlds was that I was living them all and, when each was over, I would have to pass on. It was a strange realization when reconciling my worlds that they all had that one fact in common: I had to die. Unfortunately, as a junior high student that knowledge was a little more than I could handle and only made me less certain than ever as to which world I belonged. Although it was growing infrequent, I still played tennis with a couple friends in the neighborhood, but I spent most of the rest of my time hanging out alone. I also was growing increasingly aware of the brothers and sisters I grew up with even as it became the time when all of us were going off in our own directions. It wasn't until I was out of high school, had quit college and was nearing marriage that I realized ours was a particularly blessed family.

Our quirks and troubles are the same as every other family, but my brothers' and sisters' individual characteristics had meshed into the beautiful tapestry of a family. Arlene, the oldest, always had left me in awe as a child. Eleven years older than me, she had a job at Keller drug and, as I watched her come every night, I was impressed that she was such an adult. Since then, and after a divorce, she has raised one of the most mature and level-headed young ladies I've ever met, her daughter, Kelly. Every time I think of Arlene, because of her uncontained exuberance whenever she's with our family, I think of Love.

Debby is the model mother. She talked matter-of-factly and honestly with me during my most lonely times. She has raised six of her own bright and strong children as well as two stepdaughters (one of whom, Marnie Deacon, created the cover for this book). Not just to her kids — and not just to me — but, to everyone else, she shows the best side of being a good mother, giving of herself.

David was the most free-spirited and had the greatest need to both express himself and find himself. I didn't get to know him either until we were both grown, but I always thought that he had the most creative streak of any of us kids. Eventually settling down just a little in his need to be different, David is now married with two children and has become a teacher, a job that best exemplifies his personality.

While Arlene is the embodiment of love, Jack is the most lovable. He was given the middle child role, not the strict pressure of being the oldest nor the spoiled perks of the youngest and was left to do his own thing. Jack fit in the best socially, having friends all through school. Somewhere along the line, I found it the easiest to communicate with Jack through humor. Seeing his natural use of humor helped me find my own.

Next to me, Rose was the youngest. We had little in common as kids and she, too, grew up not connected fully to anyone, resulting with her getting in with a suspect crowd that had less-than-legal reputations. But like all of us kids, Rose eventually fell in love with our family. By the time she married and had kids, she saw the need for us not to lose contact and made the most efforts to ensure we didn't drift apart. When we had grown closer together, she took it upon herself, in her own way, to watch over her kid brother. By the time I neared my twenties, one of the places I felt most comfortable and at home was with her, her husband, Paul, and their children.

While not holding the family together themselves, Harvey and Jean Burton oversaw it. Mom was the worker bee who kept a clean house, washed the clothes, cooked meals and loved to tinker at projects from re-tiling the bathroom to rearranging the furniture in the living room on, what seemed, an hourly basis. Mom was ambitious and, sometimes appearing not content to live in the deaf world, wanted to expand her horizons. She liked going out as well as entertaining at home — tea parties for her deaf friends, showers and luncheons. Whether she was teasing her brother Bud or complimenting a friend on what they'd done with their house, she felt comfortable anywhere. Enjoying travel and knowing how to entertain, she was a stark contrast to Dad. When Mom arranged plans for entertaining or planned a night out Dad, never confident in his social skills, was wary. He didn't often believe he had the power to communicate properly, yet he had opinions on every subject and when he offered one, he gave it without pretension, saying only what he truly believed. His example spoke volumes. Although he seemed to have a million rules and claimed he knew the right way to do everything, his simple manner throughout his tough life showed us kids that, if we wanted, we could be happy with whatever life dealt us. In spite of his not believing he could communicate, most of us in the family knew his love was clear.

In more ways than one, quite a bit of Harvey Burton has rubbed off on me. I, too, have an opinion on everything, I found my contentedness even when my worlds kept changing, and, like him, I grew up mostly silent and alone. When they heard that I had become an entertainer, most of our relatives were shocked that the quiet little boy they remembered as a child could actually get on stage and do a show. But that was where my father's and my lives were different. My dad's deafness and inability to communicate caused him to lose confidence in himself. When he was offered a better job than stock cutter at the paper company he worked for, he turned it down because he was afraid his inadequacies would keep him from doing a good job. On the other hand, time alone made me grow more confident. The constant talks with myself and the comparing of my worlds made me feel more alive, not more distant. Deeply believing in the power of the mind, I felt that the things hidden in it were more fascinating than any of the places one can go on this earth. I believed that I could fully experience all the things in life in my mind without having physically done so. Even though I hadn't done anything special and was only all of 15 years old, I already believed that I had led a full life.

With my feeling as if there was nothing left to accomplish in my life, I didn't think I had the need to do the things other kids my age were doing: going to football games, partying, hanging-out, forging relationships and dating. By the time I was an almost-grown adult, besides my relationship with Linda, I could count all the dates I'd had on one hand.

With 21 years of mostly being alone behind me and a growing desire to be more sociable however, I finally was confident enough to ask Cheryl to go out for a drink with me the day after we met. And with all the time I'd spent thinking on my own, I knew exactly what I wanted to talk about. I was interested in gauging where her life was coming from so, on our first date, I asked her what she thought was important in life. Possibly taken aback at such an abrupt question during a first meeting, she answered, "Well, friends, education, faith. I don't know, a lot of things." So glad that she didn't say something like, "A really cool car," I was just waiting for her to return the question and ask what I thought was important.

When she finally did, I proved myself to be a horrendous first date by saying, "Dying. You know, because everything in our life leads up to that. And since our lives are so comparatively short next to all eternity, it seems that the most important thing to focus on is what happens after we die." I was fortunate that I didn't hear the voice in Cheryl's head that perked up, looked for the waitress and said, "Check, please." I was also fortunate that she stuck the date out with me — and even went out on another.

After being unsure she wanted to get hooked up with a weirdo like me, she finally gave me another chance to not come on so strong and simply talk about our lives and what we thought about things other than death. Doing much of our courting riding around town on my Honda motorcycle, we became good friends, and, not to spoil the ending, a marriage ensued.

My conversation about death with Cheryl not only showed my views on mortality but also hinted at the faith that had grown in me since childhood. I can't remember if my parents put the idea in my head or if I just couldn't imagine a universe without a God, but from my earliest recollections, I have always felt as if I were being watched over. My version of God was not the traditional view of a long-bearded man on a throne. What I saw as God was inseparable from the air we breathed. It was a presence that I couldn't see because I was told that God was everywhere and in order to for that to be possible, I thought, He couldn't be up there wasting time on a throne; He had to be down here mixing among us. Because of constantly feeling his presence, I had the hardest time doing anything I thought was wrong. I couldn't steal or use swear words because those were the things I knew at the time were wrong and, if I did them, God would certainly see me. I even had a hard time lying because, if I were to make up some lie, the person I lied to only had to say, "Swear to God?" and I'd immediately back off, saying, "Well, no."

I don't know what it was, whether someone had put those fearful thoughts in my head or not, but I remember always feeling a presence as if someone were watching me. For years I had my own picture of the angels sitting on the floor with God watching an old RCA 15" console like the one we had in our house that stood about three and a half feet high and had wooden doors you could snap closed over the screen. After a friend in college told me that the faith I had embraced was Christianity, I delved into it further and studied the Catholic faith I was born into and eventually was confirmed at age 21. But it was the early faith that gave more depth and perspective on those days of being alone and coming to grips with dying.

Although the fall in St. Louis prepared me on a practical level for facing cancer, the fact that I had come to grips with my own death years ago meant I didn't have to do it again. By the time of my diagnosis, the thought of death was old hat. I was onto more important issues such as thinking up a new message for our answering machine. I had spent so many years mulling over, and nearly embracing, death that I was done.

There's A Method To My Trexate

It might sound like a bad joke, but there was something sick about my approach to cancer. Nobody knew it, but I enjoyed the attention. On the outside I appeared noble, not making a big deal out of it, as if I were thinking, "I've got cancer? Oh well, these things happen." Friends were impressed and fellow survivors said they wished they had such a good attitude, but I didn't deserve that kind of credit. I had spent so much of my childhood alone and unsure whether I was loved that it felt great to be nearly guaranteed that, after hearing my story, anyone other than a modern-day Scrooge would show concern.

Yet I was an adult and no longer an insecure kid. The past ten years I had connected with my family who had shared with me a love so genuine very few people get to taste it. In spite of that, the repressed longing of my youth lapped up the attention and greedily begged for more — even with the prospect of a terrible death. At 30 I was still young enough — or ignorant enough — that dying wasn't my greatest fear. I had thought about death all my life in the sense that I knew I would die *some* day. Death, since about ninth grade, had been intertwined in my every waking thought — it is what all my other fears always boil down to. But the fear wasn't immediate. Not even with cancer. I never had a sense that my life was in imminent danger. Even if I were to die, I reasoned, it wouldn't be an immediate thing. I'd have a matter of months or years, or weeks at least, and, until then, it didn't feel urgent. So, like any entertainer who gets into show business with some craving for attention, I played a cancer survivor to a caring, kind and giving audience.

It was a familiar play for attention. I did the same thing nearly 25 years earlier when I had my first life-threatening episode. When I was in first grade, I was hit by a car. I was standing on the corner of 44th and Nokomis with Kelly McGinn, a block away from school. We were walking home after playing marbles at Ericsson elementary. I paused at the corner and then, to Kelly's surprise, bolted from the curb like a sprinter. He stood there, a pale look of disbelief on his dark-skinned face, eyes widening as if he saw what was going to happen. I didn't know myself why I dashed. Not until I looked back and saw how shocked he was did I realize what I had done. And then I was shocked too.

My dash was a combination of daring, simple trust and the special kind of stupidity that came naturally to a 6-year-old-kid. Maybe I was offering a challenge to the guy in the car or maybe I was showing off. I could have sworn I had one foot on the opposite curb when I was struck, though witnesses have said otherwise. They said that when the car hit me, I catapulted across 44th street, hit a stop sign, and landed on the curb kitty corner from where I started.

It sounded worse than it was. I could have gotten right up from where I landed with little bodily harm and won $10,000 from America's Funniest Home Videos if only someone had the foresight to tape the accident. It was like a kid at a playground falling off the top of the monkey bars. After bouncing a couple of times and getting up, if there's no one watching, he'll shake off the dust and climb back up. If he sees his mother, he'll scream and wail as if he'd just been caned.

I don't know if I would have sprung right up if no one had seen me, but a crowd had already gathered because something on the sign had cut my lip and the flowing blood threw everyone into a panic. While ladies put blankets over me, I was lying on my back bawling my head off, thinking clearly to myself, "If someone would just get me a band-aid everything would be okay." I don't know if I was delirious or in shock or if I should just let the adults handle the situation. But maybe I was right. The problem wasn't that I just got hit by a car; it was that I didn't know what to do. I was confused by all the unfamiliar people and their attempts to calm me frightened me more than I already was. I just wanted to go home. Perhaps if someone would have said, "Why don't we ask him how he feels?" or "Let's put a towel on that lip and let the kid settle down," then we could have all just sat down, had some cappuccino, and discussed our feelings. But it was 1967; innocence was still alive, things were still shocking and adults believed they could solve any situation. Not only that, but espresso beans were hard to come by.

When I was loaded into the ambulance — the old kind, shaped like a hearse — I had my first realization that I was going through something special. For the moment I felt important. All those people were there for me. Since I didn't think I was in danger or even hurt very badly, it was easy to put on a brave face. What was harder was letting the hospital and my mother take care of me. I was torn between wanting their love and thinking I wasn't supposed to want it. So I relied on what I knew best, a brave face when everything else was under control. When my poor mom fainted at the hospital after I got my stitches, I walked over to her and said, "Don't worry, Ma, I'll take care of you."

I remember the weeks after the accident as some of the best days of my life because I got some of the neatest toys I'd ever had. Kids came over to our house, knocking on the door saying, "Can Scott come out?" Knowing I only had only one regular friend in the neighborhood, my mom asked them why.

"We want to look at his face."

"Go on you kids," mom said, shooing them away. "He's not a freak. He just got hit by a car." She didn't know that even though their friendship was conditional I would have happily had them in. The attention was new to me and I liked it. And the price I paid for it, I thought, was small. Years later, as I fought cancer, I subconsciously felt the same way.

After growing up being active in sports, being part of a large family in which I had to hold my own, and having parents I had trouble receiving the right kind of attention from, I had become so used to putting my brave face on that I didn't even know I was trying to draw attention to myself. Vying for attention just came naturally. I respected cancer and let people know I didn't take it lightly. But in my head, I challenged it. I was taunting cancer for show like a professional wrestler taunts his opponent in a no holds barred, loser-wears-the-weasel-suit cage match. And the attention

I got for facing cancer alone helped me keep up the act in my brain.

Although calm on the outside, inside I was standing in front of an intimidated ring announcer with a wild look in my eyes, bare chested and wearing nothing but a Speedo, screaming, "I am sick of hearing about cancer, Marty! This new Chemo guy thinks he's tough. I've made simpering babies out of tougher opponents than the masked Chemo Sabé." In the fantasy I would then look straight into the camera and point with authority, continuing, "I want you, Chemo. I want you, and, after I chew you up and spit you out, I want the Hulkster." I would then go into a flexed muscle pose.

When I went to my first oncology appointment, I kept myself from thinking what chemo would be like by picturing how well I was going to handle it. I sat across from an older gentleman in the waiting room who had the hard, tough-skinned look of one who worked the Iron Range in Northern Minnesota. After we looked each other over, he opened the conversation with the delicacy of a mid-air plane crash by saying, "So what kind of cancer you got?"

"Osteo sarcoma. How about you?"

"This is my second time."

"No kidding. Did you go through chemo both times?"

"Yep."

"Did you lose your hair?"

"Yeah. It's just starting to grow back. I was done in February."

"I'm hoping I won't lose my hair."

"Oh, you're going to lose your hair."

"That's what I hear. If it does start coming out though, I'm going to just shave my head and grow a beard out of spite." Having worked on others, that line was supposed to make him laugh. I thought he would chuckle, maybe shake his head like Dr. Thompson did and say, "You're all right kid. I like your attitude." But he didn't. He looked right in my eyes like he'd seen my type before and said, "You ain't gonna shave nothin."

"Excuse me?" I said.

He said it slower for effect, "You ain't gonna shave nothin."

There was a pause as I wondered why my act didn't work. Then he said, "You don't just lose your hair. You lose *all* your hair. Your arm hair, leg hair, eye lashes, eye brows, nose hair. You ain't shavin' nothin." After exchanging another look, we went back to reading our respective magazines.

What he said had hit me hard and I wondered if there was

something I didn't know about. For the first time I thought I might be out of my league. The game in my head, the cancer act, said no. But just as when Cheryl and I walked toward the Masonic Cancer Center on my first day of chemo, each moment felt more and more real. I didn't want to hear about my hair loss and I certainly didn't want it to be true. And if it did have to be true, I didn't want to hear it from *that* guy. Why couldn't the clinic have let me get used to the idea gradually? They could have had pictures hanging around the waiting room of Yul Brenner, Telly Savalas, Michael Jordan and Elmer Fudd. They could have sheared some sheep and let them wander through the clinic or set bowling balls in the vacant chairs, anything to help me get more comfortable with the idea of hair loss. But no. I got the message from the unaffected face of cancer itself. *"You ain't gonna shave nothin."*

Hoping I had a chance of keeping my hair and not wanting to take the word of a guy who didn't laugh at my joke, I posed the question to the nurse on my first day of chemo. Going bald was perhaps my greatest fear because it was so noticeable. It would change everything from how I looked to how others perceived me to how I perceived myself. Dying would take away my life — and I did my best to carry on in spite of that — but I feared losing all my hair would take away my humanity. And I couldn't cope with that. So I asked my second shift nurse on my first day of chemo, "Is it just a given that I'll lose my hair? Or are there some people — even one or two — who go through this and don't lose theirs?" She was polite and helpful like my first nurse, so she scanned my list of protocols. After pausing for a moment, she said, with a hint of a smile, "Yeah. You're going to be shiny." I was 0 for 2.

But by my second week in chemo, despite what the patient and nurse had said, I still had all my hair. The tough-guy act was paying off. Not only did everyone else believe I was battling cancer with hardly a hitch, I was believing it too. It didn't matter what the professionals said or what other survivors told me; I was living a movie script and movie scripts always turn out right, with the hero coming away without a scratch. People told me what could happen in chemo and I felt I understood, saying, "I'm sure anything can happen. I'll just have to wait and see then deal with it when it comes." But underneath, the voice in my head said, "Well, you see, I was a wrestler in high school. With *that* kind of training the effects of chemotherapy are nothing compared to what I've already been through."

I had an answer for everything. "You know, I almost *never* throw up. I don't know what it is about me but I don't. I didn't throw up at the Swanson's house when they made me eat that awful fish. I didn't throw up with nervousness when I had to hold pretty Mary Clemmer's hand during circle time in 4th grade. I didn't throw up swallowing a raw egg on stage once or from watching all four "Jaws" movies. I don't care what the chemo is, I just simply *don't* throw up. And my hair? Here, feel it. Give a good pull. Go on, pull as hard as you like. That is *thick* hair. Does that feel like it can just fall out? No, it's like professionally installed carpet."

To avoid the truth my thoughts didn't even have to be rational. If it came up, I was willing to say, "You know how Spiderman got his powers through a radiation mishap? I think that car accident when I was a kid did the same thing to me."

But my second week of chemo made a statement that even my best rationalizing couldn't understand. My ideas of how I'd keep my hair, not get sick and maintain my body were turned upside down during the week of what I considered to be an easy chemo, Methotrexate. I assumed it was easier because I was only in the hospital for four days and only needed a week to recover before going back in as opposed to three weeks rest between my other chemos. I thought it would be a breeze, yet whenever I mentioned to my nurses I was getting Methotrexate, they'd give out a slight, "Ooooh" and look at me as if I just told them the class bully wanted to see me after school.

I never quite got the story straight, but what I understood from my nurse was that Methotrexate had no antidote. That was alarming at first, but the nurse explained that it wasn't a big deal because there really wasn't an antidote for any chemo. "Whew!" I thought. "Now I feel a *lot* better." I took her to mean that, over the course of time, most chemos can be assimilated into the human system without damaging the person permanently. But Methotrexate couldn't be taken in slowly because in any dosage it would destroy the system. So the chemo would be pushed in over a four hour period, as opposed to throughout a whole week. For the next three days, the nurses performed what they called a rescue, in which they gave the patient drugs to heal the system that was just damaged. In Methotrexate's case it was the kidneys. To me that sounded like it was an antidote but I didn't want to argue. And I honestly didn't care. I was going to make it through anyhow.

Again I was right: Methotrexate didn't make me sick at all. I even felt like eating. I didn't tell the nurses I was hungry though because I still didn't want hospital food. So I put on another cool guy act and ordered a hot sandwich from a nearby hoagie and pizza shop. My life wasn't going to change. I would have food delivered, keep all my newspapers and half-written stories nearby on my bed and make calls on the phone to line up work for when my leg healed. It was like I was simply commuting to the hospital for work. Outwardly, I had my act together. But chemo refused to buy my act, and I didn't eat another hot hoagie for nearly two years. My brain didn't admit it, but chemo left me in a constant state of nausea. Eating that hoagie while sick made me associate that sandwich with that rotten feeling.

Interestingly, I experienced that same sickness-by-association later in chemo while watching movies. To this day I can hardly think of watching "The Rocketeer" or "Always" or "Wild Hearts Can't Be Broken" because I watched them all on the hospital in-house channel. While they are all decent movies, they literally make me sick.

I knew I would never order out again but I felt like I won that round. So I moved on to my next challenge to cancer. Since I was on top of my game and in charge of chemotherapy, I wanted to maintain my physical regimen of push-ups. While hooked up to an IV with chemo running through my body, I got down on the cold hospital floor and did 50 more pushups. Even though I was trying to be a hard-guy and in control, I should have realized how high that move rated on the Idiot-O-Meter. Looking back, I wish a nurse would have walked in on me as I was trying to be so studly.

"What are you doing?"

"Oh, I just thought I'd get some exercise in. There's no reason to lose my body any more than I have to."

"Gee, what a great idea, Scott! Pushups on a dirty hospital floor with a sterilized IV hanging from your chest. Perhaps you'd like us to re-line your room walls with asbestos wallpaper and pump in exhaust fumes while you're at it. I'm sure it'll just make you tougher."

Although I did feel a little awkward and silly while doing the push-ups, I was trying to stick to my battle plan. When I finished, I got back into bed to reclaim another part of my life by sitting down to write. Since I hadn't written anything the previous week in chemo, I didn't want to make a habit of not writing, especially with all the quiet, thoughtful time I had in the hospital. But chemo beat me to it. To my surprise I opened my book and found an entire page filled with a story. The script was almost illegible, and I didn't even think it was mine because I didn't remember taking the book out of my bag during the previous treatment. As I read the story, I finally understood what chemo, cancer and the drugs were doing to me — my body and my mind.

I stared at the page trying to place when I wrote it and what I was thinking. Above the title of the story it said, "These safety precautions, or more correctly, safety vignettes were much better than anything I could have imagined." What a bizarre thing to write, I thought. After reading the entire story, poem or whatever it was, those bizarre lines were the most sane words I had written.

This is what I wrote:
"Stories from the Core.

Little squeaky pig in bright colors and inflatable headwear
She's at the dentist's office when wham! someone gets murdered
It could be anyone, Stiff, the pixie doberman pincer who dresses in sharp all vinyl
Or the dentist, who was some over caricature of some '50s colopropult

Our one problem solvers were these little muscles and eyes
No one questioned why they didn't belong to a larger whole
Actually, I did in my dream once but I think they all had a home to go to."

Wow! I could have never known how chemo was going to lay its claim on me. I convinced myself it never would. But as I was busy building my body with exercise, protecting my job by making calls, and saving my hair through sheer willpower, along came chemo and took away my mind — maybe even my soul. Reading those lines sent a chill through my body and took away my bravado. I wasn't safe. And no amount of posturing or brave words could protect me. Forget the band-aids. Forget the medicine.

Somebody please, just hold me tight and tell me everything's going to be okay! Please take it away!

In a sense, I started my cancer journey over again when I read that story. This time, my eyes were a little wider, my expectations a little more realistic and, ironically, my heart was a little stronger. I now saw that the battle was going to be much harder than I expected. As David Byrne had said, "This ain't no party. This ain't no disco. This ain't no foolin' around." It was chemotherapy. To fight a fast-growing cancer. My life *was* going to change in ways I couldn't imagine, but I could at least prepare for and maybe even accept the change — *if* I wasn't so stubborn.

I started by embracing the story that knocked me off my feet, reading it over and over again and sharing it with others. It fascinated me that I had no recollection of writing it. Reading it was like watching a National Geographic special about some neurological disorder: "After cultivating and sowing his 100 acre cornfield, farmer Dave Mahoney of Dublinville, Iowa, who suffers from Chemo-itis Dementia, wakes up the next morning forgetting all the work he'd done the previous day and begins to plant oregano."

About a month after writing it, I was working on a fledgling radio show with some other comics, and I couldn't resist having some fun with them. We were at the home of Ken Bradley and Colleen Kruse, working with Steve Matuzak, a comic book/story writer. Gathered around the dining room table, we had stalled in our writing when the conversation turned to how I was doing with my chemo. "You want to know what chemo's like?" I said, almost daring them. I had just had my revelation of what the treatments were really doing to me and was eager to share that with them. Not knowing what to expect, perhaps wondering if I was going to give them a regurgitating visual, they simply said, "Sure."

"This is what I wrote my second week in chemo," I said baiting them slightly. I knew they expected something serious, so I played into the drama. "It's called "Stories From The Core.' I have no idea why. But this is really what my mind was like while on chemo." My friends looked at me blankly, not knowing what to expect. Then I started, "Little squeaky pig with bright colors and inflatable headwear." Colleen was the first to burst out laughing and none of us stopped until the story was finished. "What's really bizarre," I told them between the laughter, "is I wouldn't have written any of this in my book unless I was thinking, 'Hey, this is *great* stuff! I can use this in my show sometime.'"

And I have done it at a few shows. The first line leaves the audience stunned as if they just don't get the joke. But as I continue, they catch on that the joke is in just how wild the story is. I don't even perform it for laughs; I just love telling it. This is how the rest of the bit goes:

"She's at the dentist's office, when, wham, someone gets murdered. *At this point, some ex-druggie chimes in, 'Oh wow man, I know how this ends.'*

"It could be anyone, Stiff, the pixie doberman pincer who dresses in sharp, all vinyl. *I can't explain that line too well, but I think it's some type of reference to the Gap. It is, however, notable that, in my mind, 'Stiff' was a pretty good name for a dog.*

"Or the dentist, who was some over caricature of some '50's colopropult. *Now those of you playing along may have noticed that 'colopropult' isn't a word. But, fortunately, being a word isn't a criterion for getting into this story.*

"Our one problem solvers were these little muscles and eyes. No one questioned why they didn't belong to a larger whole. Actually I did in my dream once, but I think they all had a home to go to."

Closing the book I say, "That's what it's like on chemo," and let the audience digest it however they can. When I finished that last line for the comics, however, Colleen said, "I like that part." And so do I; it feels almost poetic. It's for the sake of those last lines that I wished I could tap into what my mind saw, what I truly meant. But those words will remain an artifact, a fossil representing the mystery of my mind on chemotherapy. Cheryl, who has been a poet for the past 10 years, says she can't figure out the meaning. She has said more than once though, "That's the best stuff you've ever written." I think it was a compliment.

I finished the week of chemo physically and follically intact, but my sense of being and my perceptions were shaken. No longer would I issue a challenge to chemo. Chemo issued one to me, the challenge of surviving.

But, like a wise-cracking uncle who tells some lie and, when you say "Really?" he screams "Gotcha!" chemo had one last eye-opening prank to leave me with that week. When the four days were over, my primary nurse, Michelle, who was one of the best at talking to me like a real person, sat me down on the bed and went through the checkout procedure with me. It was all standard stuff:

watch my temperature, clean the catheter tube and get all my things together. Then she handed me some pills and told me I had to take one every six hours for three days.

"Why?" I asked, since I didn't have medication after my last chemo. Michelle maintained her comfortable, matter-of-fact tone, as if she were simply reciting a step-by-step list of how to apply bathroom tile grout, and told me I needed the pills to keep fighting Methotrexate's poisoning effects. Those pills would do the job at home.

The situation sounded serious, and I wanted to know how serious it was, so I asked, "What happens if I don't take the pills?"

"You'll die."

"I'll die?" I thought. "Just like that? I'll die?" She said it so casually. To me, this sound like a bit of a problem: Taking pills every six hours so I don't die! For the first time in the hospital I *didn't* want the nurse to treat me like a mature human being. I wanted her to treat me like a helpless two-year-old. I wanted her to say, "Well that's okay wittle Scotty Wotty Botty. You can stay wif us and we'll help you get aaall better. We'll give you your wittle pill evewy time the teeny hand on mister kwock moves six numbers and all you have to do is take a big dwinkums of water. Isn't that nice, hmmm? Who loves his auntie Michelle?"

I didn't feel right asking them to treat me like a slobbering infant so instead I said, "Well, if they're that important why am I leaving the hospital?"

"We trust you."

"But I can be sort of a forgetful person sometimes. What if I forget to take one?"

"You won't."

"But really, what if just once I happen to…"

Her voice slowed and became deliberate so that I understood both words clearly: "You *won't*."

I paused for a moment, looking at her.

"You *won't*," she said once more.

And I didn't.

You've Got What?!

After two rounds of chemo and three months in and out of the hospital, I occasionally had to explain to people why I wasn't working much or why I seemed to have dropped out of society. When a friend who did some promotional work for me in 1991, in exchange for my doing a show for him, called to book me for his Halloween party, I awkwardly replied, "Um, I don't think I can. I'm in the middle of chemotherapy."

"Oh," he said, as if I'd just told him, "Sorry I can't make it. I'm dead and this is a recording." I felt bad that he hadn't heard about my illness so I offered to do a show for him when my therapies were over. He regrouped quickly and agreed that maybe I could perform some other time. But both of us knew that the other time could be never.

I didn't have to tell many people the news before I gathered there was no correct way to tell others about having cancer. Because of the horrible stigmas associated with cancer, most people expected a little drama. For them, listening to my diagnosis was like watching a man on death row waiting for an 11th hour call from the Governor. Their faces hung sullen with concern and fear as a spectacled, Radar O'Reilly-looking county clerk receives the call. His eyes widen with the urgency his responsibility bears, and with sweat on his upper lip and forehead, he tears down the death row corridor. The sweep hand on the clock rounds 11:59. Click click

click go the clerk's heels, echoing down the hallway. With fifteen seconds left until midnight, the sweep hand presses on as all eyes stare at the clock. When the clerk bursts through the execution room door, all heads turn expectantly towards him. He takes a couple panting breaths, pauses, then says, "It's cancer."

Besides a couple of distant friends, the only person I remember telling was my sister Rose. That's how fast news spreads in my family. My sisters are pretty good at dishing gossip, but my mom has made it an art form. The woman could have worked for the Pony Express without a horse. I've told my mom about important shows I was leaving town to do, and by the time I got home there were three messages on my answering machine wishing me good luck from distant relatives in upstate New York whose last names I don't even know. She has known personal information about me before I knew it myself. Many times she just blurts out bad news, but usually Mom's pretty good at delivering information in a socially accepted, melodramatic way. With Rose being the only one to give the bad news to, I just hoped whoever told the rest of the family about my cancer did it in a tactful way.

I was never one for high drama, and Cheryl wasn't either. Neither of us knew exactly what it meant to have cancer, but that was all the more reason not to make more of it than it was. So by the time we got to Rose's, we were feeling playful and not in a telling-your-family-you-have-cancer mood. "Man, look at all these kids," I said when we got there. She had two of her own that weren't in school along with our three. "You should get yourself a couple sheep dogs to keep 'em all together."

After Cheryl went to say hi to the kids, Rose and I talked in the kitchen. "What did the doctor say?" Rose asked, wanting to get to the heart of the matter. "I'm not sure," I said, trying to keep the conversation light, "but I think one of the interns was the same guy I saw on a wanted poster at the post office." Rose made it clear that she didn't want to hear jokes; she wanted to know what my diagnosis was. "They're not exactly sure," I said, "but they think it's an osteo sarcoma."

Rose didn't say a word. She's not an outwardly emotional person so I couldn't tell what was going on in her head. I got the impression that she accepted the news much the same as if I'd told her I had diabetes or a heart murmur, afraid for me but not torn apart. No one in our family is overly emotional, so I expected that response from everybody. Rose's silence was uncomfortable to me because I didn't know where she stood. Was she okay with it? Was she scared? Did she think I was going to die? I spoke up, wanting to set her at ease that both Cheryl and I accepted it — at least as much as we knew about it. "We're okay with it. There's really not a whole lot we can do except take whatever comes. I mean what else *can* we do?" I paused hoping that would make sense, even if it wasn't reassuring.

"You know what I'm doing?" I asked, not giving Rose a chance to answer because it would have taken way too many guesses anyway. "There's a line in the R.E.M. song 'Me In Honey' that I'm embracing to help keep perspective on this whole thing." Then I sung the line to her, "Let me lo-ove, what it's doin' to me." I knew that cancer could change my life, but that line helped me think I could love the change and that I could love my life just as much with or without cancer.

After I sang those words, Rose lifted her hand to her face and cried. At first, because I rarely sing out loud to my family, I thought I must have sung so poorly she was laughing. The next second I realized my words weren't comforting, because she was crying. She cried so hard, her entire body was shaking, and I was shocked to see her like that.

Maybe her emotions had been building up for the past couple of weeks since my biopsy. Maybe hearing her little brother tell her he had cancer was the last straw. Maybe she loved me and didn't want to see me suffer. Or maybe I was so emotionally crippled that type of empathy was foreign to me. Whatever it was, Rose's tears, like Cheryl expressing her fear before my allograph, brought me back to reality. Not only did I have cancer, but I had an entire family whose brother and son had cancer, a wife whose husband had cancer, children whose dad had cancer and good friends whose pal had cancer. I had the disease but we all suffered.

Not that I ever read it, but there was a book out a few years before my experience called "Why Bad Things Happen To Good People" that applied to our situation. I was tempted to investigate it, but I ultimately concluded it was one of those questions that didn't concern me. It's not that I thought bad things *should* happen to good people or that I wasn't a good person, but I've read the papers and watched the nightly news. I know about World War II, discrimination, natural catastrophe and countless other examples of human suffering. I've known all my life that bad things didn't just happen to good people. They are available to us all — and usually for free.

There have always been books that have asked essentially the same question — C.S. Lewis' "The Problem Of Pain," Phillip Yancy's "Disappointment with God," even the book of Job in the Bible. Job, himself the embodiment of a good man suffering, asked the question. As I recall, God answered all relative inquiries when, in verses of eloquent poetry, he told Job, more or less, to shut up. I didn't want a book to explain it to me anyhow because why bad things happen isn't a question that can be answered with a pat explanation. I believed it had to be lived and discovered for oneself.

It didn't take cancer for me to realize that bad things have to occur to all of us in life. I never wanted to admit it, but not knowing one person who has never had a bad stroke of luck plus having no verifiable proof of Shangri-la indicated that struggle is just another part of life. Even after getting cancer, I never felt I had authority to argue that bad things shouldn't happen. I had been and continued to be content letting God have sovereignty over that problem. I do know, though, if bad things *never* happened to good people it would sure be easier to spot the rotten people in the world. "Hmmm, look at Johnson over there. He just got over chronic bowel control loss; now he's suffering from dry, flaky skin and hair loss. What a jerk!"

But suffering at least on some level, I've always thought, is simply part of life. When I was about 15 years old, I had a recurring vision of the entire planet, not unlike the picture I had of Debby pushing me in a wheelchair along a small arc of earth. I used to lie on the wooded, grassy hill leading down to Lake Hiawatha near my house, and seeing the trees, lake and thick grass all around, I imagined nothing but forest and green plants covering the whole earth. No streets, cars or even houses, just the natural growth of nature if man never existed. That was the most beautiful vision I've ever had of our planet, existing in perfect harmony like an empty, lush forest. I knew then that the earth in that state was as close to perfection as it could ever be. When I think of why there is suffering, I only have to imagine a handful of human beings dropped down into that peaceful ecosystem to stake their claims, and that would be the perfect recipe for trouble.

Perhaps the greatest stumbling block to asking why bad things happen to good people was, to do so, meant I qualified as a good person. I want to believe that I am, but who is or isn't a good person is subjective anyhow. For all I know, years ago in the midst of a burning hot sandstorm in central Mongolia, Genghis Khan was debating the same question. While plotting to rule the world, he might have been sitting in his tent in tremendous pain, suffering from a really bad case of athlete's foot. He could have been there itching and scratching his toes like mad, soaking his feet for hours and walking gingerly.

Perhaps Genghis turned to his chief advisor, who was busy tallying up how many people they had slaughtered that day, and screamed out, "Why does this always happen to me?! *Nobody* should have to suffer like this. I mean I'm a nice guy, aren't I? I'm very social, always out there meeting people, trying to make fair deals. I've worked hard to get where I am today. I could have gone the easy route and taken that job with the accounting firm, but no, I'm following my heart. I'm being true to something I believe in. And then (pointing to his wretched feet) *this* happens. Why me? Where is the justice!?" Although most people would probably conclude that Genghis doesn't qualify as a good person, the rest of us have our own gray areas. Too gray for me to judge anyhow.

What made my suffering worse than dealing with my own pains and fears was there were all sorts of other people that I considered good who had to suffer along with me. I didn't have the right to question their suffering, but I felt — and many other survivors I've talked with agree — that the struggle with cancer was harder for those who loved me than for myself. Even though I suffered the physical pains of my leg and the tiring chemo, it was a pain I could grasp. There was a real presence I could struggle with. The pain of my cancer was a one-on-one battle where sometimes I was on top and sometimes cancer was. But there was comfort in being able to see the battle. It was *my* battle.

My poor family though could only watch from the outside. They didn't know how I felt and they only saw how I looked, hooked up to an IV and thinning. They only knew the awful stories that said if you have cancer you're going to die. They couldn't be sure I was even *in* the battle. Not knowing tore at them mentally, spiritually and even physically. The bottom line was they were helpless. And that's the worst way to be: To look into the face of pain — even death — and know there is absolutely nothing you can do about it.

When Rose cried, I realized cancer would affect others in ways I couldn't imagine or control. Like adapting to having cancer, I eventually had to adapt to people reacting to my cancer. It became a strangely reciprocal relationship where I had to treat others with the same helpless pity with which they treated me. As with Rose, I felt awful that I couldn't do anything to help her from feeling bad about what was happening to me. It was a vicious circle.

Perhaps his caring advisor felt the same pity for poor Genghis. "Oh Decimator of Civilization," he might have said, "I feel the great pain you must be suffering. If only it were my pain to endure. I would take away for you the damnable curse of cracked, itchy skin." Then, feeling the same way I did, Genghis may have said, "Ah, but who am I to complain. You've been tallying up the countless victims for days now. You are generous to be concerned, but they are my feet to worry about. When we destroy Switzerland, I'll buy you some chocolate."

In time, the circle alternated between vicious and endearing. How a person reacted to my predicament was a barometer, directly proportionate to how much they cared, or feared, or were confused by my cancer. There were some who truly cared, such as Cheryl, who faced my situation with complete assurance. The reactions reflected the scope of human nature: shy, melodramatic, uninformed, even the know-it-all response. No reaction I received seemed inappropriate. In our parents' living room Arlene said, "I suppose I'm going to have to get used to saying the 'C' word."

"You mean cabbage?" I asked.

Ken Bradley, one of the comics who I worked with on the radio show, told me his first reaction to my having cancer was, "Oh no. Who's going to mow his lawn?"

Once, in the middle of my therapy, after chemo had ravaged me physically, I ran into one of my friends at a comedy club. He was a young, well-known comic in the Minneapolis area with whom I had a professional relationship, performing occasionally together on the road or at local clubs. I was on crutches, pale, thin and bald, and my brother and I had just finished watching the comedy trio The Higgins Boys and Gruber. We were heading toward the elevator when we ran into my friend.

He didn't even recognize me. When I said hi he stopped in shock, his eyes growing nearly larger than his entire head and looking completely aghast. "Scott! I ... I don't know what to say,"

he said, as if he thought my death were imminent. "I … I …" he
went on to say. "I … don't know what to say," he repeated. The
comic part of me wanted to then fall to my knees wheezing,
coughing and gasping for air screaming, "Quick, Heimlich me!"
But having seen the debilitating effects cancer had on people, it
would have been far too cruel, even for a fellow comic. Instead I
told him everything was fine. I assured him I didn't expect to die
soon and that I hoped to perform again. From his blank stare, I
guessed he believed me.

The people I saw every day grew used to my look. Like anything
shocking — violence in the movies or when men first started
wearing earrings and dresses — my look eventually grew commonplace. But whether my story was accepted or treated with fear,
I became thankful that people cared. My look gave me an open door
to talk about what I was going through — and others listened. If I
looked completely normal others may not have had the patience to
hear my story at all. So cancer and the look it gave me provided the
opportunity to communicate my words, my heart, my life, my*self* to
anyone who would listen.

Strangely, that was a perk. It is something we all can use, in
sickness and in health: The freedom to speak most fully and deeply
our minds and hearts. What a joy it was at that time to have an open
forum to laugh, cry, wonder, to be utterly confused, ask stupid
questions, orate and express my complete humanness. That joy
was almost worth the disease.

And maybe that's why bad things happen to good people — so
we have a chance to communicate. Perhaps we need things to go
wrong in our lives so that we can turn to someone else, someone we
love, and ask, "Why?" If everything were perfect in our lives, if
nothing ever went wrong, what reason would we ever have to
share our lives with other people? When the world seems like an
ocean of sinking souls, it's a little easier to reach out and to ask for
help. Perhaps we're supposed to muddle through just so we can
rely on each other.

I'd always loved communicating anyhow. Being on stage,
trying to teach my mother how to pronounce the word *soldier*,
arguing with David about the nature of reality — it all filled me with
joy to pass on my ideas. Although it might have been another way
of drawing attention to myself, communicating was my constant
source of joy. With cancer I not only got to communicate and

exchange ideas, but I also got to be taken seriously. Being in my profession, and having a history of joking too much, I could have appeared to my family as if I were pulling a prolonged, ill-conceived gag. "Okay, Scott, that's real cute. Ha ha ha, you had cancer. Now, before you offend someone, quit messing around, unhook that IV and get out of that cot."

All of a sudden, cancer allowed me to be taken seriously. I didn't have to try to be funny, and my family could see that I wasn't joking my way through life. They looked into my eyes and I looked into theirs and, whether I was being silly or deeply honest, everything we said acknowledged, "Yes, I do have cancer. This is what I look like. I do plan to keep on living. And yes, the world is still okay."

The only person besides Cheryl who didn't seem to look at me with fear throughout my cancer episode was Jack. He was the person who I joked the most with — so much so, he seemed to be one of the few people that understood that my joking was a response to how serious and afraid I was. I didn't get to see him much during my cancer experience. He had been living in L.A. for the past five years and only got to visit a couple times. (Once he was flown out by the comedian Louie Anderson, a friend of mine. Having influential friends like Louie was another perk I had as a performer.) Although we talked infrequently, our discussions always felt even-handed, sometimes philosophical, sometimes metaphysical, often making fun of the world. With or without cancer, I could always count on Jack to be, in the truest sense, brotherly.

Jack never pulled any punches. I remember years ago when I wasn't as conspicuous at getting attention, I tried to do a little emotion baiting on him and he didn't budge then either. Jack and Rose were in the kitchen of my parents' house. I was whining about losing the marginal body I had as a high school athlete and was looking for cheap affirmation. Complaining about the unstoppable growth of my waistline, I said, "Man, I'm just getting so fat." Rose, bless her heart, was about to counter with the kind of stroke I was looking for, saying something like, "Are you kidding?" That was when Jack put down the paper he was trying to read and with perfect timing said, "No kidding, Porkchop."

With Jack as his personal advisor, I think I'd even feel sorry for poor Genghis.

You Say "Potato,"
I Say "You're Bald"

I had countless issues to debate in my head while fighting cancer. Part of me, for example, wanted to eat healthy, while the other part decided that since I already had cancer, I might as well eat whatever I felt like. Part of me wanted to take it easy and let my body heal while the other part wanted to run rampant, exercise and do tricks on my crutches. But, while there were always at least two sides to every situation in handling life with cancer, the issue that polarized my logic against my emotions the most was the probable loss of my hair.

"It's inevitable. My hair is going to fall out."

"Oh no it's not. It's staying right where it is."

"How can you say that? You heard what the nurse said. You read the pamphlets. Remember that guy in the clinic? It's *going* to happen."

"It's not going to happen. Hair doesn't just simply *fall* out."

"It does when you're on chemotherapy."

"Does not."

"Does so."

"Listen, I don't need your negative energy, man. You always look on the dark side of things. I know who I am. I know my body. I know my hair."

"You *know* your hair? You're talking like a crazy person.

Chemotherapy, by it's design, destroys all fast growing cells in the body. That means it attacks cancer cells, but since hair follicles are fast growing cells, you and I both know they have to go too."

"All right mister, wise guy know-it-all. I'm sick of your pathetic outlook. I'm sick of being in this ridiculous situation and having you prattle on about accepting all of this. Let's go. You and me right now. I'll kick your candy-ass butt all over this floor, you whiny livered, disease infested, bad attituded sissy boy."

"Oh yeah?! You want a piece of me? You want a piece of this, you future bald headed, gimp-legged, vegetarian, no-brained, can't-accept-reality moron? Come on, I'll clean your chemo-in-fested clock."

Internal arguments and debating were not new to me. Before I ever had cancer, making any decision was an intensive process. Every issue involved going through checks and balances in my head as I questioned the procedure of everything from how to make a sandwich to mowing the lawn.

The seemingly simple matter of how I was going to drive to a show meant I had to go over what route I would take again and again. "If I take the highway, I'll be going out of my way," I'd think, "but if I don't make the lights on Lake Street, I'll waste just as much time," I'd answer. "And do I even want to get there so early?" I'd go on, apparently enjoying the conversation. "Why not take my time," I'd think, assuring myself. "That way I can go over my show and listen to my favorite songs on the Innocence Mission tape."

It wasn't that I felt pressured to make the best possible choice as much as I liked knowing why I did what I did — regardless of how trivial it seemed. My system of nit-picking over everything was my form of obsessiveness, but growing up with five other kids who endlessly questioned or mocked each action of their siblings ingrained the habit in me.

With cancer, I finally had a cause worthy of being obsessive about. Before my ordeal, when I was caught up in day to day living, my inner turmoil was mundane. "Do I watch 'Seinfeld' or tape it?" "Should I do the crossword or the word jumble first?" "Original recipe or Extra Crispy?" When I got cancer, the non-stop questioning of my every move actually seemed appropriate. From taking pills to cleaning my Hickman catheter to doctor appointments, everything I questioned was centered on my staying alive. Maybe cancer was God's way of accommodating me.

The fact remained, however, that my issue-wrestling du jour of losing my hair was a fruitless one because, after all was said and done, whatever was going to happen would happen. If my hair was going to fall out it would no matter how good of an argument I put up. I saw losing my hair as a step toward losing my humanity. Maybe it was not wanting to be treated differently or be seen as being sick that kept my fear of going bald looming over my cancer experience. Or maybe it was vanity. But no matter how much I tried to avoid it, once I lost my hair I would officially be a cancer patient. "So what," the smart-alecky know-it-all side of my brain chimed in. "Nothing can take your humanity from you. You can only give it up yourself. If you act like a human, you'll be treated like a human, no matter what you look like." The belligerent side of my brain, not having a good answer, fought back, "Yeah? Well I think you're stupid, a lousy dresser — and it really smells on your side of the skull."

As much as I feared the absence of my personhood and of others treating me differently, by being a man, hair loss wasn't that extraordinary: A man losing his hair was less likely to be treated as a shock than a woman going through the same thing. I couldn't imagine what going bald would do to a woman's self-esteem. Do women act like balding men, I wondered. When a woman's hair falls out does she buy a little red sports car and start dating younger men? Does she start hanging out at bars and asking everyone to call her "Cindy?" I knew that a woman's hair greatly affected her self-esteem. My mom dyed her hair, curled it, teased it and styled it every way possible. From the moment it started turning gray, until she was sure it was all the same color, she wore a wig. My sisters, too, always fussed over their hair. So by the time I started chemo, the idea of a woman losing her hair was like a man being emasculated.

On Masonic 3, I saw a woman after her hair loss talking in the halls about how well she thought she was handling chemo. "You know, in a few years there'll be chemos that don't even make you sick," she said in a voice well acquainted with local bars and VFW halls. "But I don't care," she went on. "I got through my last chemo and I'll get through this one. All I need to do is get up and walk around every once in a while. I'll be fine." With a scarf wrapped around her head, she didn't pay any attention to her scalp or people's reactions. When I passed her, she looked right in my eyes without an ounce of self-consciousness. I was impressed. "If that woman can come to grips with hair loss," I thought, "she can deal with anything life threw at her." Seeing her and other women, totally at ease with chemo baldness helped me be less conscious of my own.

"Okay okay," the less accepting side of my brain mildy conceded. "What if, and I'm just saying *if*, what if my hair were to come out? It wouldn't be so bad if it fell out gradually. I mean, are we talking elderly gentleman slowly balding or an autumn gust of wind blowing leaves out of a tree?"

"We're talking big avalanche in the Rockies," replied the other side confidently.

"Oh my. Well, it could be a relief I guess, if it all fell at once to get it over with. That way I wouldn't find hair all over the place. That is if it *were* to fall out."

"Oh, it's falling out. Trust me."

"Is not."

"Is so."

"Shut up."

"You shut up."

"I don't have to listen to any of this."

"This is the way I see it happening," the accepting side teases, as the other half says to itself in a sing-songy voice, "I'm not listening ... "

"You and me, by virtue of sharing the same head, are out at some restaurant with Scott's wife, Cheryl. We'll take two bites of food, have a drink of water then boom. We'll look down and it'll seem like we're eating a Pekinese."

The other side of the brain begins plugging its ears and whistling. "How do we explain that one?" the winning half continues. "Uh, waiter. There's a wig in my soup."

All the debating, arguing and worrying did little more than occupy my time. Yet the inner turmoil was important because it helped me get comfortable with how I fought cancer. No decision I made about my care was necessarily the *right* decision; it was just right for me at the time. And it was only right for me because I took the time to find an answer. Because I took that time, I believed in what I was doing which was the most crucial element in beating cancer. I was an active participant. The issues were comparatively small — losing my hair, what to eat, how to exercise — when set against times when my life was in imminent danger, like later, between chemos, when I caught a blood infection and my body went into uncontrollable shakes. Debating about my future, more or less, kept me in practice so that when it came to protecting my life, decisions were quite easy.

There were a million ways to look at every one of our problems, and I was comfortable with that. The only thing I took exception to was when other people came to tell us *their* ways to solve *our* problems. When I was first diagnosed for example, a woman came over and told us the miracles of a proper diet and the importance of cleansing the intestinal system. Later a man gave us a video tape about his high-protein shakes and vitamin pills. And to top it off, toward the end of chemo, a salesman who looked like a 90-year-old Pat Morita came to our house and unfolded an industrial strength futon, telling us that sleeping right would keep us healthy forever. From the comfort of my own couch, I reasoned that all the possible remedies used in tandem could very well cure mankind of all known diseases, but they weren't for me because, at the time, I only knew how to believe in my doctor and chemotherapy. So that was what I did.

The remedies everyone offered me gave me the choice of *how* I wanted to live while fighting cancer, but my greatest concern was *that* I got to live. Although I wrestled with it, the question of how I wanted to remove the tumor wasn't that big of a deal. Dr. Thompson gave me the choice of either a plastic knee, of fusing the joint which would leave my leg locked straight, or the cadaverous allograph that I eventually went with. That fusing the joint was even an option was hilarious to me. Given the choice, how many people would be thinking, "Yeah, that straight, peg-legged step has always appealed to me. As a matter of fact, why don't we fuse my elbows and lock them up as well. I could get a job at a road construction site telling cars to slow down." I figured fusing the joint became an option because it was the cheapest. All the hospital needed was a huge spot-welding machine.

Aside from the no-contest on fusion, the decision between the plastic knee, which supposedly would be replaced every 10-15 years, or the bone transplant was worth considering. But which choice was *right* was a moot point since neither one was a life or death decision. Dr. Thompson never posed the question, "Well Scott, you have this high grade tumor in your leg that will soon spread and ultimately kill you. What do you think? Should we leave it in there or take it out?"

"Hmmmm, let me see ... "

The most important decisions were the ones about which I had the fewest choices. When it came to diet, for example, I had a whole spectrum to chose from. When I had my blood infection, however, the options were to go to the hospital or die. After Methotrexate, my choices were to take the pills every six hours or die. In those matters, there wasn't a whole lot of debating going on.

Choosing the allograph was a foregone conclusion anyhow since I knew that was what Dr. Thompson wanted. He talked it up more than the other options and spoke often of its lasting power and my prospects for a long life. The doctors let me believe that I made the final decision, but Cheryl thought they set us up. In her eyes, when Dr. Thompson and the med students gave us the options, it was as if all these white coats and stethoscopes were gathered in a semi-circle around us with gleeful looks saying, "Well Mr. Burton, you can have the *allograph*," as the doctors all nod along approvingly, flashing car salesmen smiles and a neon applause sign lights up above their heads while the Mormon Tabernacle Choir sings the Hallelujah Chorus in the background.

"Or," they say, as the room darkens and their heads all move closer while they put flashlights to their chins and make menacing faces, "you can have the **PLASTIC KNEE JOINT**." The music from the "Psycho" shower scene plays, and they shake their heads disapprovingly while one of them fakes a heart attack. Either decision was fine with me. Heck, I would have even gone with the fused knee joint if that were the only way to keep my life.

Across the board, life has always been the easiest choice to make. Once, while sharing ordeals with an elderly woman who was also a cancer survivor, I told her of the high-tech, cutting edge surgery I had, and she said what others usually pointed out. "Well, at least you got to keep your leg." "If it was a matter of remaining alive," I said, "They could've taken the leg. As far as I'm concerned, they could've taken everything from the neck down. I'd still be able to think, breathe and share my life with friends. Besides I wouldn't take up much space, and I'd be guaranteed a spot on all the major talk shows."

As for what I was going to do about my hair, nature and medicine finally made the decision for me. It happened so quickly, as if a switch was flipped in my scalp to make my hair begin dropping out in bunches. I was home one evening between chemos. Due to the pain and hassle of trying to sleep upstairs in our bed, I was sleeping on the couch. As nonchalantly as I had always done, I ran my fingers through my hair. For the first time ever, a clump of hair went along with my fingers rather than staying on my head where I usually kept it. I didn't feel it come off though and wouldn't have even known it if I hadn't felt a small amount of fur in my left hand. I looked at my hand and, not making the connection, thought, "Now that's the darndest thing. We don't have a dog."

Once I made the connection, I got on my crutches and went into the bathroom to throw the hair out and take a look at the bald patch that it left. Oddly, I couldn't find one. Since other cancer patients and nurses had told me about the nuisance hair loss becomes — showing up in food, clothes, bed and numerous other places where I'd rather not have clumps of hair — I found a scarf, wrapped it around my head and went to bed.

Although I checked all week long, I never found where any of my hair had fallen from. (As nearly as I could tell, it seemed to be coming from somewhere in the vicinity of my head.) Hair was all over the place, yet when I looked at myself in the mirror, my head looked as normal as it always did. I was like one of those hair-growing Barbie Dolls where you just keep pulling and pulling and hair keeps coming out from the deep recesses of her empty cranium.

What struck me as even more unusual was that it didn't hurt when my hair came out. I had always associated pulling a fistful of hair from my head with a certain amount of pain, but I felt nothing. I did have a constant, itchy, slightly burning sensation all over my scalp, but when I pulled on the hair, there was no feeling at all. It was like the numb feeling of Novocain when I got my wisdom teeth removed or the first time I wore a steel-toed boot and asked everyone to stomp on my foot. The positive side was I felt no pain. But on the negative side, I felt no pain. Normally, the absence of pain is a good thing, but I felt losing a major part of my head should include some physical recognition of it. Sure it didn't hurt, but like a leper losing a digit, I was losing my hair and didn't even know it.

I took advantage of the good news angle of no pain by occasionally making it a performance. A few weeks after my first chemo, my family — Rose, her husband Paul, Dave, his wife Amy, Arlene, our parents and I — were sitting around the kitchen table of my parents' house. I was wearing the bright red hat Dave had bought for me, the one with a black and white spiral insignia on the front that looked like a hypnotist's eye-catching trinket. He had bought one for himself and my dad as a sign of kinship between us. It was a kind gesture, but for me, the hat said, "Well, if you hadn't noticed that this guy's hair is falling out yet, at least check out the goofy red hat he's wearing."

Rose asked why I was wearing the hat and I casually replied, "Because I think my hair's starting to fall out." Dave asked why I thought that. So I took off my cap and, in the same manner that you'd offer someone a stick of gum, pulled a lock of hair out and showed it to him. It reminded me of a spoof Saturday Night Live did some 20 years ago called the Nuclear Family, about a family that lived near Three Mile Island whose bodies mutated until their hair fell out regularly. But I didn't have writers or supporting cast. Mine was real-life, not a spoof.

To their credit, my family didn't react with an "Oh my goodness," which, as a showman, I was going for. They responded with a cavalier "Oh," as if they saw that kind of thing every day. I threw the hair in the garbage and did a couple more performances to show that the first example wasn't a fluke and I felt no pain in de-hairing. Dave was the first to state the obvious: "Why don't you just cut it all off now?"

"Cut it off!?" the unaccepting side of my brain screamed. "Why that no good ... Let me at 'em." While half of my brain wanted to jump out and have it out with Dave, my more sane side realized that my family had actually gotten ahead of me in accepting my chemo side-effects. I was supposed to be the one saying to them, "Well, I hope you can get used to looking at me without any hair," not them saying to me, "Aw, come on, Scott. Don't be so sentimental. Your hair never looked that good to begin with." I was a little stunned and only answered Dave's suggestion of cutting it off by saying, "I don't think so." Yet they all just kept looking at me as if I were being obstinate, their faces saying, "Well, okay. It's *your* head."

Although I knew cutting my hair made perfect sense, I couldn't bring myself to actually do it. I couldn't adequately explain why except to say, "Because it's my *hair*. One doesn't normally do that. 'Let's see, what do I have to do today? I need to pick up some groceries, stop at the post office, take the car in, shave my head skin bald, write my parents ... "

Cutting all my hair off because it was bound to fall out anyhow had that same illogical ring to it as tying my shoes when I'd just have to untie them later. Or getting ice cold because it feels so good to warm up again. Those examples, though, were weak analogies compared to what I faced. Mowing all my hair off before it fell out felt more like saying, "Well, ultimately, I'm going to die anyhow, so why not bury myself now to save time?" Hair is just one of those things a person tries to keep as long as they can. Ask any guy who combs his seven locks of hair from the left side of his head all the way over to the right. My hair looked so much better on my head than in the wastebasket.

I kept an obstinate attitude for about another week, and true to what other cancer patients had told me, I found hair everywhere. It was in my bed, on my clothing and all over the house. But since I still couldn't find any clear patches on my head from where the hair came, I remained in denial. As long as I didn't wake up one morning and find a perfectly molded wig of hair on the pillow, I could still believe I wasn't going bald. Without seeing white patches on my scalp, I almost convinced myself that there was no concrete evidence that it actually was *my* hair that was all over the place. There was plenty of circumstantial evidence to support the case, but I refused to be swayed.

Finally, a couple weeks after my second chemo, the itchiness got to be more than I could handle. To satisfy my urge to scratch, I stepped out our back door with a wire brush, bent over and brushed my hair wildly. So much hair came out I couldn't clean the brush out fast enough. It was like the thick, matted hair we used to get when brushing our dog. Part of me was delighted with the fun of it all while the other part was thinking, "Gee, this can't be a good sign."

I finished only after satisfying my itch and went to the bathroom to search my scalp. Looking in the mirror and lifting up my still fairly thick hair, I saw a gaping patch of white. The gig was up. To not admit my hair loss now was like trying to innocently tell my mom I didn't eat any of her cake even though I had chocolate frosting all around my mouth and a butter knife in my hand. I couldn't deny it any longer. Both sides of my brain came to an agreement and admitted that my hair would be taking an extended leave of absence. The formerly disagreeable side even said, "If it's going to go, and I know it's going to go, what the heck, why not throw it a party?"

I showed up at Dave's house with a red cap and a full head of hair. He supplied the clippers and Jack Daniels. (Actually there was no liquor involved, though, in hindsight, that may not have been a bad idea.) I'm happy to say Dave had a good time. The first thing he did was give me a mohawk. Dave buzzed the rest of it off, and then, as I was feeling the tiny stubble on my skull, went on to say, "You know I think this should be a bit shorter." "Yeah," I said. "Perhaps going down a couple layers of epidermis would be good."

He was right though. He found another attachment — I think it was from his vacuum cleaner — and took off another 1/8 to 1/4 inch. Satisfied the job was done, I began taking off the towel from around my neck. But Dave, being a rather fussy sort about fashion, said, "Let's trim this up over here." In my head I'm thinking, "Trim?! I don't think there's any trimming left." But I was in no position to argue. He seemed to be enjoying himself, was doing a good job, and was wielding a razor.

It was actually pretty sweet. I was looking only for the hair to be removed by any means necessary. I had no illusions of coming out looking better than I did when I went in. If an old butcher knife was all we had to do the job, then that's what we'd use. My brother took it more seriously. I only expected a standard military buzz cut, but instead I got a trip to Ché Dave.

And it looked pretty good. As good as if I were simply someone looking for a radical change in my life and thought shaving my head was the way to do it. Dave, being the kind of person who would do just that, agreed. There were a few skin patches from where my hair had completely fallen out amongst the shady dark stubble that gave my head the geographical look of a map of the Middle East. But those patches where helpful because, if anyone asked what I'd done to my hair, I could tell them it was a political statement. As much as I didn't want to put my red cap back on to cover my baldness, I did. It was a natural reaction. Intellectually, I felt as if I was covering up my cancer. But I knew that was physically impossible.

I drove home afraid of how my family, most importantly Cheryl, would react to the new me. She, of course, was wonderful. Just as she had accepted my cancer and dealt with my disabling surgery, she told me my head didn't look all that bad. I knew she was being honest because she didn't use words to make me feel better, placate me or humor me. If she would have said, "Gee, honey, you look great! I hardly noticed a difference," I would have known she was playing a game. Saying it didn't look too bad said she expected a lot worse. My look was like a stain on the tablecloth or clothes that didn't quite match. Baldness wouldn't have been her choice, but she could deal with it. Growing to find it beautiful took time and a unique grace that was Cheryl's special gift.

After Cheryl made me feel comfortable, the kids gave their complete and unabridged opinions. I didn't expect acceptance from them, but I got it anyway in Rachel and Dylan's first responses. Matthew was only a year-and-a-half old and was too young to be outwardly affected. (We've noticed, though, that he has a strong fascination with touching and wearing hats. Maybe *that's* his response.) Rachel and Dylan acted squirrelly when I got home which they always did when something new was brought into their lives. They hid, ran around the table, played silly word games and giggled incessantly. Rachel, when she felt more settled down and comfortable, was the first to comment on my new do. In typical Rachel fashion she said, "Dad, you sound the same but you sure look different."

I smiled and gave her a hug. Her five-year-old honesty was exactly what I needed to hear to know I was still a human. So I pushed the issue a little further. "Do you like it?" She didn't need to think about it but she waited a moment, perhaps to spare my feelings, and said, "No. I don't like it as much. But it's okay. If it was the medicine that made it happen that's okay because it's going to make you better." I didn't have the heart to say to her, "It wasn't the medicine that did this. It was your stinking Uncle Dave."

Dylan, too, responded in his own unique way. No one ever knew what to expect from him. Our next door neighbor, Margaret, used to say, "Dylan is more himself than any child I know. He doesn't try to act like anyone else. He's just so ... Dylan." So anything he said would have been normal. And yet his response still seemed to come out of left field. He was three years old at the time, and as we were in our dining room sitting at the table, he sheepishly said to me, "Dad?"

"Yes, Dylan."

"Take off your hat."

I could rationalize why I shouldn't feel strange taking my hat off, especially in front of my own son. But it was my first day and I was still trying to get accustomed to it.

"Naw, I really don't feel like taking my hat off, Dylan."

He got a little more persistent and, with Spanky McFarlane cuteness, said, "Da-ad. Take off your hat."

If he weren't my son I probably wouldn't have done it. He was acting so darn cute and I knew I was going to have to get used to doing it sometime, so I figured it wasn't a big deal?

"All right, Dyl."

When I took my hat off, Dylan's shoulders hunched up to his neck. His eyes crinkled and sparkled behind his long dark lashes as he put his little hand up to his mouth and let out the most delicious giggle I'd ever heard from him.

The kid set me up! My three year old son set me up! I'm currently looking at brochures for military schools.

I was fortunate to get a few more strokes like Cheryl had given me and a couple more like Rachel and, luckily, no more like Dylan's. With the inner battle over, the whole hair thing grew less important. It became apparent that my hair was the last thing I needed to worry about, which was a good conclusion. Because one more argument with myself over my hair falling out and I know I would have kicked my butt.

My Problems, My Roommates and The Near-Wonders of Attivan

"What could possibly be my motivation to go in for chemo again?" I asked Cheryl before making my third trip to Masonic 3. I was ornery, tired and not at all happy with what it had done to my hair. "It's not like, since last time I was there, they've invented a new and improved chemo that's easier to ingest and leaves my mouth with a fresh minty aftertaste. There is no 'Chemo Lite — a third less nauseating.' Why would I want to go back?"

"Maybe so you don't die?"

"Oh yeah. Good point."

Cheryl was even less enthralled with chemo than I was. Believing in a holistic, natural approach to cancer, she would have let me quit treatment at any time, but since she knew I had accepted chemo, she encouraged me to stay with it. "I'm amazed that you're already on your third treatment," she said. "In a way it's going fast and in a way it's not. Like, when I'm home with the kids while you're gone, after it's over it seems so distant, but while it's happening it seems to last forever." "Yeah, it's weird," I agreed. "I still have that feeling that it's all a surreal dream, a test of some kind, and any second a game show host is going to jump out and say, 'Well, Scott, I'm sorry you didn't do so well in the chemo round. You were supposed to complete that round without throwing up.'"

But we both knew it wasn't a game, so we got into our car and headed to the University once more. Although I'm not in the habit of quoting philosophers, a line of Friedrich Nietzsche's helped me look on the positive side of chemo: "That which does not kill me makes me stronger." (I did question the line a little. Nietzsche obviously didn't intend for that line to be used in every circumstance — after all, he's dead.)

Although the staff usually wanted me on the floor by 9 a.m., I didn't arrive at Masonic 3 until about 10 that morning. Being late was my own quiet rebellion for chemo not being ready before sundown. I wanted to do *something* to let them know I didn't like waiting around for nothing, but I never had the guts to call them from home and say, "Listen, I'll be in when the chemo is there, ready and waiting for *me*." I'm not a confrontational person though; I entertain thoughts of creating conflict, but I'd feel terrible if I ever followed through with them. Instead of being a pompous jerk, I make jokes, complain to Cheryl, or stew about my problems. I should have my own commercial on late-night television: "I'm not only the president of the Passive/Aggressive Club for Men. I'm also a member."

On that particular morning I confronted my morning nurse in the best way I knew how, "So what do you think the problem is with the chemo this week? Maybe they were having a big party down in the pharmacy and they used all my chemo for the punch?" She smiled. "It could be," she said with a hint of a laugh. "But sometimes," she repeated once more as if there were cue cards in the room, "it takes a while to get the orders written up and the chemicals mixed downstairs."

I can see now that my constant questions about the delay of the chemo could have been annoying, but the nurses didn't mind. They were kind, talkative and willing to laugh, even when I couldn't let that issue go. Not once did they say, "Man, what a jerk you are. No other patients are complaining. Why don't you quit whining and be glad you *don't* have chemo." It's possible of course that they did — just not around me. As much as I don't want to wear on people by making jokes, maybe when I thought I was being inoffensive, the nurses were all back at the station saying to each other, "You go in. If I go in I might knock him upside the head with a bed pan."

Aside from not wanting to hurt their feelings, I tried not to be offensive because I knew the nurses weren't the ones who mixed my chemo. They only hooked me up. What good would it do to lay into my nurse when all she could do was call down to the pharmacy where an amoeba-like, slow-bodied druggist would say, "Scott still doesn't have his chemo? Gee, that's too bad"? These people were too decent to dump on.

Besides, I knew there must be some reason for the day-long wait for chemo, even if only God, the FDA and some sadistic practical joker down in the lab knew what it was. Not to mention, if I were to exercise an offensive rebellion, the nurses held the trump card by having the last say in administering my chemo. "Let's see Mr. Prima Donna Burton who comes in whenever he darn well pleases, I think the orders for this round of chemo to run through your veins calls for a half bottle of tobasco sauce. Mmmm. That's going to be tasty."

While the most frustrating problem was the tardiness of my medicine, it was only one of many that plagued me upon my checking in. Before I even got to my room to find the chemo wasn't ready, I had already endured the first indignation of returning for treatments — the odor. The terrible hospital/chemo smell on Masonic 3 was a debilitating aroma that wafted throughout the floor like flatulence on a muggy day. Strangely, Cheryl hardly noticed it, but the moment the elevator doors opened, that smell hit me like driving through Iowa farm country with the windows down. Powerful enough to make my knees buckle, the smell made me wish I were in a car so I could roll the windows up.

Each time I crossed the threshold of the floor, my gag reflexes tightened like a cat coughing up fur balls. "Was everyone just so used to the smell," I wondered, "or was it only disgusting to me because I was taking chemo?" If it wasn't just me, how could anyone on the floor be satisfied with that terrible odor? Why didn't they do something? Even students in the most rank college dorm room, buried in fermenting sweat socks, rotting pizza cartons and stale beer go through the futile effort of hanging up one of those pine tree air fresheners. How could no one have linked the wretched smell on Masonic 3 to the problem solving agents of air freshening products? Have the multi-million dollar marketing efforts of Glade been entirely for naught?! Often after chemo, I had wanted to visit my nurses, but decided to stay away for the same reason that, as a kid, I stayed out of the kitchen when my mother gave one of her friends a perm.

Yet because I've been in other hospitals and on other cancer floors without noticing a similar horrible stench, perhaps the odor wasn't due to chemo after all. Maybe it was a terrible odor unique only to Masonic 3. Perhaps one of the nurses had some cream cheese and herring for lunch back in 1953 and no one had thought to throw it out. Maybe some of the interns had a gas problem. Whatever the reason, whether it was the chemo or some other mysterious source, that rancid odor was a problem for me.

When I finally managed to get past the gauntlet of odors and drab halls, I made it to my room but, being a veteran of chemo, I knew that right on my heels would come a nurse's assistant pushing along a scale and carrying a thermometer kit. It was far less of an annoyance than waiting for chemo or a rude odor, but for some reason it was imperative to chart my girth and body temperature the minute I reached my room. It was as if getting the chemo drugs to begin therapy could wait, but waist and inseam measurements had to be taken immediately.

At the time I didn't understand at all. Taking my temperature was something my mom did when I was trying to get out of school and weighing myself was something I did when I got out of the shower. How did those two things become scientific criteria for saving my life in chemo? Weight and temperature seemed so inconsequential, so non-medicinal that I figured the hospital's next step for treating my cancer would be placing a nice cold wash rag on my forehead. Not until over a year after getting out of chemo did I learn that my weight and temperature when I arrived at the hospital were crucial factors to mixing chemo.

But from the beginning, I believed the key to getting through chemo — like the key to being a good juggler, both on and off stage — was having a good attitude. Life on Masonic 3 was filled with annoyances, but there was still something endearing about it. I enjoyed trying to make the best of a bad situation. Although I was in a cancer ward, I was still able to smile, and because I honestly enjoyed the staff, I wanted to share that with them. So when the guy came in my room to get my weight and temperature that week, I approached it like a comedy routine. I looked at him and said, "You know this is a good idea." He was a good natured sort, a little slow but bright-eyed, so he smiled at me and said, "Oh yeah?"

"Yeah," I said, "When my wife and I have guests over for dinner we tell them, 'Dinner will be ready in about an hour. In the meantime come on upstairs to the bathroom so we can get your blood pressure and a urine sample.'" As he smiled again, I added, "You'd be surprised how willing they are."

The wild card that disrupted my good attitude was the drugs I was given to cope with chemo. Benadryl, Compazine and Marinol were some of the many medicines the staff offered me. During my first week, I was given Zofran, which was widely considered a miracle drug. Zofran was the one drug that could slow, sometimes even halt, nausea with no side effects. On my first day in chemo, I heard one woman in the hall saying that when she had chemo years ago, she could hardly even stand up. "This time around, with Zofran," she said, "I hardly feel a thing. Now if only they had a drug that let me keep my hair," she quipped, "I'd have it made."

Aware of the fate of Elvis and Howard Hughes, I preferred to take as few medicines as possible. Besides, if there was a singular miracle drug for nausea, that suited me just fine. Just as I was persuaded by Dr. Thompson's pitch about the bone transplant, I probably would have taken Zofran even if it hadn't been a miracle drug because of the huge marketing blitz behind it. Everyone was talking about it, nurses, sur-vivors, and even the doctors. Because of insurance influences and not wanting to be biased, doctors didn't always talk about specific drugs. But Zofran was different; they went on about its virtues, praising its existence like high school girls gathering before gym class talking about their current crushes. "Well, Jenny in 3rd period is using a syrupy kind of drug with a lot of side effects. But I 'm in love with Zofran. It's *dreamy*."

I was given Zofran my first week along with a number of other drugs from the pharmaceutical palette. Strangely, after both doses of Zofran, I felt a tightness in my chest and a little shortness of breath. "Nobody," the staff guaranteed me, "has ever reacted to Zofran." But to their credit they checked me out thoroughly and even hooked me up to a big machine that went "ping." They were dumbfounded as to what the problem was even though I kept telling them, "Well, it seemed to start after I took the Zofran." A succession of two nurses, a doctor and a couple heart monitor technicians all said they had never seen a reaction to Zofran and stopped just short of saying, "Well, maybe there's just something wrong with *you*."

And maybe there was something wrong with me, but I still wanted the tight feeling in my chest to go away. Perhaps it was only nerves from my first day in chemo, but until I knew what it was, I asked for something other than Zofran. That, in hindsight, was not a good move.

Some patients, when they direct their own medical care, are impeccable in their judgments and have even helped heal themselves. I, on the other hand, made my medical judgments the way a carny at the State Fair guesses your weight — no science, no real knowledge, just a seemingly random lucky feeling. My consistency for being wrong would be a Vegas pit-boss's dream. Right or wrong though, I felt a patient should make his or her best effort to understand and be active in the therapy. Being part of the decision, I was better able to accept any circumstance because I was involved in my therapy. And I thanked the staff for trusting me in making decisions. I also assumed that they wouldn't let me make any that could seriously harm me:

"Gee, these electrical plates sure seem interesting. They just go right here on my chest?"

"Clear!"

Pfffffft.

In the absence of Zofran, the nurses gave me an alternate drug called Attivan. Instead of fighting nausea, Attivan was a strong relaxant, a sleep-inducing drug. Although Attivan wouldn't prevent me from vomiting, it did help me forget the vast amounts of vomiting I had already done. As an amnesia inducer though, it also helped me forget the people who visited me, what was on TV, which day of therapy it was and, sometimes, who I was. Though forgetting large chunks of my day wasn't in my plan, Attivan could make me feel like I had slept over 24 hours a day, which was a great benefit when I was in a hurry for the week to go by.

Although Attivan didn't work that way every day, my lack of retention caused problems for those who came to visit me. And Cheryl got the worst of it. My poor wife was struggling to keep a household together, pay bills, watch kids and maintain her sanity, and still she made it three times or more a week to visit me. But due to the near wonders of Attivan, I often didn't even know she had been there. Once, when my mom visited, I asked her, "How come Cheryl never comes to see me?" My not remembering amused my friends because, since I appeared alert and made jokes, they thought I was doing fine. Then, when they learned I didn't know they had visited, they'd either not believe it, marvel at the potency of the drugs or feel sorry for me all over again. But they didn't have to invest as much in maintaining a visiting schedule or be a single parent, so they were rarely offended. Unless she felt good just to get away or didn't care if I remembered anything, there was no payoff for Cheryl's visits. That she did visit so often and that I recognized it so little says her coming was more of a kindness than any regular hospital visit. After all, if she didn't want to visit, she could have easily hired one of the visiting South American interns to enter my room and pretend they were her. "Ayllo, Scote. Theez eez Charil. I ope you are feeling goodly. I weel see you again so soon."

"Thanks for coming, dear. Say hi to the kids."

Strangely, while Attivan kept me from remembering parts of my day and visits, I still had some vivid recollections of my roommates. Not all of my roommates because I didn't talk to all of them. Sometimes, because of the curtain between our beds, I didn't even see some of them. Not knowing whether they felt like talking and afraid to make the first move, I rarely started conversation. Consequently, I was left to refer to the ones who didn't talk as the loud screaming guy, the coughing guy and the sleeping guy.

My first roommate, Rex, would have rather not talked to me at all. But on that first day of chemo, I was chatting like the new guy in the office trying to make friends. "How long have you been here?" "Are you scared?" "Where do you live?" "You're not going to be throwing any parties over there are you?" Intimidated by the ominous surroundings of an unadorned floor, the smell of chemo and a guy living on the other side of my room, I talked mostly to figure out the rules of the place. Was I supposed to introduce myself or would every patient rather be left alone?

From the nurses tending to his needs I learned a little about him. Besides overhearing his name, I pieced together that he not only had Lymphoma, but had lost his sight and some fingers to diabetes. Eventually, enough awkward time passed with both of us knowing each other was in the room so that no matter what we would have said it would have felt forced. I finally had to say something. "Hi. I'm Scott." Trying to fill any awkward gaps, I jumped in before he answered. "I gather you're Rex."

"Yeah. Hi."

"I hope you don't mind sharing a room," I said, looking for anything to say besides, "I'm so terribly sorry you have cancer."

"No, I don't mind. If you don't mind me playing my radio."

"No, I sure don't," I replied when, in fact, I did because it was always on and was too loud. But I would have let him do anything because I felt so awful for him — blindness, amputations *and* cancer. I was too immature at the time to understand that, yes it was terrible but, many cancer survivors — or survivors of anything — have accepted what was dealt them and move on. For some reason I treated him the same way I didn't want others to treat me.

We didn't talk again until the next day when I entered the room while he was eating. Although he was blind, he certainly knew I was there as I watched him with his finger in his pudding cup to know how much he had left. I hate small talk, but felt again like something needed to be said. "I'm amazed you can stomach the food. I really haven't been able to eat a thing since I've been here." He told me chemo hadn't affected his appetite. As the conversation went on, he opened up a little more and we talked about our experiences. He was a minister with a wife and two kids.

I was happy to know he had a family that loved him, but deep down I still pitied his situation. When I finally got the nerve to ask about his blindness, he said, in a distant, matter-of-fact way, "When I was a kid, I had diabetes. I never took care of it. My brother had it too, but he took his insulin and watched what he ate. I didn't care. I was acting like a kid, doing whatever I wanted, eating candy like I was getting away with something." His voice trailed off, just wanting a chance to go back in time, knowing that childish act had defined his life. He seemed aware he couldn't have it back and that was, somehow, okay.

Rex declined when I asked if he wanted me to read to him, and I made a few more feeble attempts to start a conversation. But I don't think he ever considered me a friend, which was probably fair because I don't know whether I was actually being a friend or merely trying to make myself not feel so bad. After leaving that week, I almost wished I could have had another shot at being friends with Rex. But we never connected again.

I put my patronizing attitude on hold when I spoke with Tony, the next roommate I conversed with. Tony and I met during my second chemo, after I'd learned I couldn't mend anybody's heart or attitude. All I could do was listen and, for Tony, that was enough. A native of the Iron Ranges of Northern Minnesota, he was a massive man with a gentle heart. As with Rex, he was already on Masonic 3 when I arrived, but, unlike Rex, he started our conversation. After I was settled in and had my weight, temperature and a blood sample taken, Tony asked about my cancer the same way he might ask his drinking pals guys about hunting deer up north. "How are you doing? Is this your first time here? How long you staying?" We traded questions and I told him my story, trying to get him to smile or laugh, telling him about the guy in the clinic who said I was going to be hairless, about my visits, about juggling and wanting to love my life in chemo. Then I asked him his story.

Hearing him talk, like a scared boy sometimes, sometimes like a quiet philosopher in the shell of professional wrestler, I was struck and humbled by the kindness in his voice, the heaviness in his heart and the power of his will. As he spoke, there was no agenda to his story. He told me honestly and sincerely what he had been through, about the cancer growing in his back, how the doctors couldn't get to it, the pain he was going through at every step, about it seeming like there wasn't much time left for him. He said all of these things without looking for pity, as if telling the story over and over again would help him understand the sense of it all. It was as if he believed that telling the story one more time might help him find an answer.

Tony was the only patient in chemo who felt like a friend. We only had the one chemo round together, but it was enough to make me want to keep hearing his story and share mine. I felt honored that, although his pain was nearly insurmountable, even for as large a man as Tony, he still wanted to talk to me. I was angry at the doctors for allowing his pain to be there. There must have been something they could have done. Yet to think I could fix his pains or make him feel better like I tried with Rex seemed foolish.

For Tony, just talking made him feel good in spite of the pain — talking and listening to my story. How could I even try to ask how bad it hurt or suggest he try lying on his side more? He was the one living it, I was on the outside. Instead I listened because it seemed that's what he wanted me to do, simply be there. Listening to his stories I said "wow" so many times I sounded like a doped up college kid listening to a theory on parallel universes. I wanted to recommend Dr. Thompson to Tony and help him find out more.

But Tony already knew more about dealing with cancer than I did, and Dr. Thompson didn't do backs. Besides, his talking had such a therapeutic quality that for me to have given my opinion would have taken away the magic. During my next chemo, Tony and I were being treated at the same time, but in separate rooms.

And when I was done that week, I left without saying good-bye. I don't know what I was thinking.

Because I hardly talked to any except the last one, I remember the rest of my roommates by their sounds, their visitors or their smells. I distinctly remember the guy who came in after Tony though I didn't talk to him once. He was so deliberate and assured in everything he did. I watched him like I was watching someone else's home movies, commenting to myself on his every move. "Who *is* this guy? What is he doing now? Why does he act like he owns the place?" He and his wife came onto the cancer floor, into my room and more or less took charge. Perhaps he was a business-man who was used to taking control. A little guy with short gray wavy hair, a body like Joe Pesci's and a pinkie ring, he began barking at the nursing staff about his plans as if he were staying overnight at a Bed and Breakfast and expected a lo-cal, high energy chemo shake first thing in the morning.

Even though he didn't talk to his wife even once, she confidently supported him as he commandeered the room. Appearing to be in her late fifties, she also emanated that rich version of being dolled up: a fur coat, evening gown-ish clothes, lots of jewelry, make-up, a dark wrinkly tan and that kind of aerosol sprayed hair that you can throw a rock at and not mess up. If watching these two was like watching someone else's movies, at least it wasn't boring. When he first came in, I was amused, thinking, "I'll bet this is his first chemo. Boy, is he in for a big surprise." Then he began discussing his chemo plans with the nurse. "Fat chance, fella," I was thinking. "You'll be lucky to have your chemo before the Vernal Equinox."

Although the Rich Guy initially entertained me, he quickly left me enraged. In the middle of bantering with the nurses, he walked over to the thermostat and turned down the heat. I couldn't believe it. As far as I was concerned, patients simply didn't do that. By messing with the thermostat he changed me from a voyeur into an unwilling participant. And not only that but an angry one: I had been cold every day in chemo, even during the previous week. Before rooming with him, I often kept the door closed to keep the heat in and always felt bad asking for more blankets since I already had two. I wanted nothing more than to walk over and turn the heat up all week, but I assumed the staff didn't want me playing with it.

So when that guy went over and turned it *down*, of all things, I wanted to scream out, "Hey! Hey! Hey! I *live* here, pal! I don't go over to your house and switch the channels when you're watching TV do I?" Remaining true to my passive/aggressive nature, not one word passed my vocal chords, but I was livid. In my own home when I was growing up, the thermostat was the ultimate taboo, so I just assumed that law would be the same in the hospital. Any second I was waiting for my father to walk in, take a look at the thermostat and yell out, "Okay, who's been playing with the heat? Do *you* want to pay the bills?" My pointing finger was all ready.

Still not having said a thing — but having had several conversations in my mind — I leered at him as he walked back and began discussing his routine again. Never quite saying anything, I mulled over what I could say to make him feel bad for what he'd done. Maybe it was the drugs or because I was out of practice, but the best zinger I could come up with in my flustered state was, "Hey, you big dumb head!" Meanwhile, having found out his chemo wasn't going to be ready on time ("Surprise! Ha ha ha!"), he casually mentioned to the nurse that he and his wife would be going out for dinner. Going out for dinner?! I couldn't believe what I was hearing. " I hope your spit tray overflows," I thought.

Maybe that's what I was most angry about, that I hadn't done anything. Even after everyone had left the room, I *still* didn't have the nerve to get out of my bed and turn up the thermostat. For all of my wanting to be a part of my treatment, here was a classic case of my doing absolutely nothing.

My brain started mocking *me* at that point. "I tell ya, you don't want to mess with Scott Burton, no sir. Don't get me riled up. Don't get on *my* bad side, boy! 'Cause, if you do, why I'm liable to just go ahead and sit around and *stew*. I'm not afraid." Fortunately the near-wonders of Attivan kicked in and, within ten minutes, I was asleep and forgot about the episode for the rest of the week.

Amazing Grace

As another week rolled by and my cancer fight was a couple months old, problems mounted concerning every facet of my treatment. I was having trouble ingesting Methotrexate, I'd been back in the hospital between chemos with a fever, my bone graft wasn't healing well and both my body and brain were feeling the tiring toll of therapy. All of that and that guy messing around with my thermostat to boot. I had, it seemed, a perpetual font of things to whine about, yet, when asked how the fight was going, I'd usually reply with some version of "Can't complain."

But I *did* complain — to everybody. I complained about my leg not healing. I complained about the number of blankets on my bed. I complained about what was on TV at night. Usually with jokes or an accommodating smile, so it might not have seemed like whining, I complained about whatever I could. It was hard to tell, though, whether I was complaining specifically and sincerely about my slow progress in chemo or if I was just being my usual self. I've spent over half of my life complaining or at least commenting on everything I see and I was no different during chemo. As a comic, complaining is my job: I can't help but endlessly point out absurdities, if possible making them funny. I try to think of it as an affectionate running commentary on life, but for anyone who has to hear it all the time, I'm sure it comes off as one big gripe.

Unfortunately for Cheryl, she's had to be that one person. While eating dinner at an upscale restaurant once, I was curious why the caesar salad had a fishy flavor I'd never tasted before, so I asked the waitress if there was fish in the dressing. She said there was and that anchovy is a key ingredient in any good caesar dressing. Still reeling from its potency, I leaned to the waitress and said, "I'm not sure, but I think there's a little bullhead in this one." Another time, when ordering pizza, I was told it would take an hour to get it delivered. Not thinking of it as a complaint, I instinctively blurted out, "Whoa. What? Is there a convention in town? The Shriners all called at once?"

Both the waitress and the pizza guy laughed partly because neither line was delivered mean-spiritedly. But Cheryl, being present both times, just gave me a sly look and a smile that said, "You know, I've heard all those jokes before. And even though everyone thinks they're cute, you're really just whining again." And she was right. Whether they laughed or not, whether they smiled or enjoyed my company, and even if I was trying to be kind, I was still — if only a little — complaining.

I've often tried to rationalize my nit-picking. "The way I see it," I told Cheryl, "Nothing can ever be perfect. So pointing out flaws is facing reality. And that helps me strive for what, ideally, is better." Cheryl gave me a dry look that said, "I've heard that line before too." "What you're asking," she said, "is for everyone else to live by your ideals."

And I knew she was partly right. For example, when Rachel was five, I expected her to clear the dinner table with the efficiency of a veteran waitress. My own ideals can be as unnatural as man-made lakes — they look good and sound good but, in the end, are something created for my own convenience. "But there is still a perfect ideal somewhere," I pleaded, "an ideal our very universe is structured on." Cheryl said nothing, but gave a look of, "Hmmm?" knowing neither of us could prove what I just said. She agreed but was suspicious whether I — or anyone — could be the one to know exactly what that ideal is. While accepting it and being a little intrigued by it, Cheryl sees my commenting on everything as more of an obsessive bloodletting, a complete inability to let anything go.

Pointing out the negative side is as deeply ingrained in my family as politics is in the Kennedy's. And, while their obsession pays better, ours is something nobody in my family is spared from. Once, when Cheryl and I were getting ready for our third anniversary, she was wearing a new wool dress by Norma Kamali. She was gorgeous, hair wildly curled and just a hint of make-up. Everyone else raved about how she looked yet the first thing my mom said when she entered the room, pointing to Cheryl's nose, was, "Oh, you got a pimple there."

It's so sad. The last thing my mom wanted to do was make Cheryl self-conscious on her anniversary night, but it is such an immediate reaction for all my family, she couldn't even help it. So Cheryl was right about my negative nature, but it's not as if I invented it all on my own.

The way I look at it, this negative approach has a built-in positive side. I contend that loving the world when everything goes wrong is at least as important as loving the world when everything goes right. That was the philosophy that kept me loving life throughout cancer. If I could find laughter — and share laughter — about the difficult side of life, what was wrong with that? It was my way of acknowledging that the world is an untamed beast. Yet I know the difference between laughing and loving life when tough times come, as opposed to bringing hard times upon myself. With my disease, however, I didn't have to look because the difficult times came to me. So when I joked and complained, it didn't sound like obsessive whining; it sounded like fighting cancer. Even to Cheryl.

Still there were times when, no matter how hard I looked, even I couldn't find a thing to complain about. There were some things I couldn't comment on or joke about. There were times when all I could see was joy. I could only stand with my arms limp at my side in wonder, awe and simple gratitude. Those were the times when I knew how outrageously blessed I was: Debby taking me for a ride in the wheelchair, my nurse setting me at ease before chemo, the success of my operation and my family truly loving me were all blessings that, in a sense, dropped out of the sky. They humbled me, filled me, and I had no control over them. They came to me when I could never expect them, sweet gifts from God.

While each blessing was as sweet as rebirth, the most astounding, humbling and life-giving blessing was that Cheryl still considered me attractive. I was sunken and hollow-eyed, sickly, thin and hairless. Yet not only did she say it often, the look in her eyes said she still thought I was a beautiful man.

Finding me attractive was the icing on the cake. There was nothing that could have prepared Cheryl for sticking with me through all the ups and downs of cancer, much less loving me while doing it. She was raised in a disconnected family. Hers was the kind of house where no one talked around the dinner table and there were certain perceptions of what a person was supposed to do: take swimming, tennis and piano lessons, don't talk back, do chores, speak when you're spoken to, send thank-you notes, smile when guests are over, go to college and don't marry until you've got a career. If she followed all the rules, she was assured, life would go on without any problems. When things went wrong, it was not uncommon for it to be hushed up or not talked about openly. Yet all that Cheryl had expected in life and was trained for got turned on its ear: she didn't finish college, she married at 21, her husband didn't finish chores, she had three children who *did* talk back and didn't write thank-you notes *and* her little-bit-lazy husband had cancer.

Adapting to the disarray we were thrown into was the exact opposite of what Cheryl had grown up with. My expectations had always been high, but knowing her life, even Mr. I-expect-every-thing didn't expect her to take on every responsibility. She not only managed to embrace every turn in my therapy and recovery; she did it as if she had been doing that kind of thing all her life. She communicated and listened, showing me the kind of kinship every survivor needs. When friends called to offer her support, she supported them. When the kids needed a mom, she was there. When my family tried to muscle in on my care, she battled them. And when Dr. Thompson called her about my biopsy, she was crestfallen. But there was something that made her look each problem straight in the eye. Even when she looked at cancer, she wasn't afraid. Somehow she was able to see beauty and life. She saw the rest of our years together and all our years before. That was when I knew who was truly blessed.

I tried a few times to view myself as attractive. I'd look in the mirror, open my mind and think like someone who'd never seen me with hair, but all I ever saw looking back at me was E.T.'s homely brother. To cope, I went back to joking. Sitting around my parents' kitchen table, I held up one of the last remaining hairs on my arm and said to my mom, "You see that? Once that hair is gone I no longer qualify as a mammal. I'm going to have to apply for amphibian citizenship." Before that, during the third week in chemo, "People" magazine's annual cover of the Sexiest Man Alive had just come out. On the phone with my dear friend, Judy, I bragged that I was voted the Sexiest Man in Chemo. "It was a close race," I said, "and actually I was only the first runner-up but was eventually declared the winner when the judges found that the guy who won was only an old mannequin they found in storage and not an actual living chemo patient."

Jokes and reassessing my self image, however, could only take me so far. Without Cheryl's unconditional support all my jokes would have been hollow. She not only found me attractive but treated me, looked at me and spoke to me as if I were a beautiful man.

Without hesitation and more than anyone, Cheryl accepted me, even when that meant accepting the possibility of my death. Her acceptance opened the door for all my other blessings. And because of that *she* was my greatest blessing. While I joked, complained and looked like a horror movie extra, to her I was beautiful. But it wasn't, "Well, he's my husband and I have to pretend I'm not affected by his looks." Although not considering me a double for Robert Redford, she was attracted to me. I was so hung up by my looks at the time that I didn't see the obvious: She loved me.

When asked where her strength came from, her drive and her peace, Cheryl said throughout our entire episode and even afterwards, that she was given a special grace. Just hearing her mention that word made me feel warm because it fit her so well. Her grace was so obvious, but not everybody knew what to call it. In his book "Wishful Thinking A Theological ABC," Frederick Buechner summed up what I loved so much about the word. Here is his definition of Grace:

> *After centuries of handling and mishandling, most religious words have become so shopworn nobody's much interested anymore. Not so with grace, or some reason. Mysteriously, even derivatives like gracious and graceful still have some of the bloom left.*
>
> *Grace is something you can never get but can only be given. There's no way to earn it or deserve it or bring it about any more than you can deserve the taste of raspberries and cream or earn good looks or bring about your own birth. A good sleep is grace and so are good dreams. Most tears are grace. Some body loving you is grace. Loving somebody is grace.*

Grace was Cheryl's blessing. She had the grace to laugh along with me instead of cry, to, without warning, become a single mother to three small children, to watch our finances dwindle and still trust in our future. She was even quoted in the newspaper as saying, "I'm excited to see what we can handle." Who else could look at all that had fallen in our lives and say, "I'm excited"? And the bonus to her being under the veil of grace meant I shared the same veil.

And she shared mine: My joking, love of life and nit-picking attitude rubbed off on her after eight years of marriage. Sometimes I got on her nerves and she'd tell me to quit whining. Other times she thought I was in denial, to which I'd look her straight in the eye and say, "No I'm not." She made jokes with me and even made jokes of her own when I was depressed. Once, as I considered whether my lifestyle had contributed to the disease, I said aloud, close to despair, "Man, I'm just a young, goofy looking, worrying buffoon." Cheryl coyly chimed in, "Honey, don't say things like that." Then with a sparkling hint of a smile she added, "You're not that young."

At 5' 4", barely 100 pounds, Cheryl is the kind of woman most people would call petite. The third time we went out, I casually mentioned, "You're such a petite thing." I was trying to tell her that her small size combined with her high cheek bones, strong jaw line, long brown, naturally curly hair and deep, hypnotizing blue eyes made her one of the most uniquely beautiful women I'd ever met. But that's not how she took it. Without even looking at me, she said with a quiet forcefulness, "I may be small but I'm not weak." I instantly believed her and said, "Uh, yeah. I'll *bet* you're not weak."

But contrary to her guarded statement, I was drawn to her. Her quiet manner, honest faith and her soft and innocent voice attracted me. I remember being close to her, walking around Lake of the Isles thinking her quality must have been written in stone before she was even born. Her quality was and always would be sweetness.

Unfortunately Cheryl doesn't agree with that now. Twelve years of marriage to a guy who's idea of sweet is a well timed burp accustomed her to my less-than-tactful approach to life. Actually she was buried in a similar bluntness by my entire family. Everyone in my family is outspoken. We not only say what's on our minds, but we're prepared to spend hours backing up our points, poring over every detail until we have worn the other person out. Though we've softened since Cheryl and I have been married, no one in my family has been afraid to make bold statements, lay themselves on the line or resort to sarcasm. For Cheryl to adapt to such a verbose and argumentative family called for a 180 degree switch from her upbringing. And regardless of whether we blame our feisty manner on having deaf parents or our need to control or wanting attention in a large family, from Cheryl's perspective it was either stand her ground or be eaten by the wolves.

In her own way, Cheryl followed suit. Sometimes she spoke her mind on the spot. Other times she stewed about it, talked with me, then got mad and had it out with whoever offended her. Either way she got into the mix — laughing, teasing and speaking her mind. Having adapted to our thrust and parry version of social interaction, Cheryl believes she's changed into a crass, opinionated woman. That she thinks this amazes me. Anyone who meets her recognizes immediately that she is simply a beautiful woman steeped in a warm brand of sweetness. Even ten years with the Burton family hasn't made her hard.

Yet Cheryl couldn't help but second-guess herself, in her nature and how she presented herself to others. Throughout my cancer she didn't fret about outward appearance anymore, and that was part of her grace. But she was frustrated and second-guessed herself because she was thrown into a position where she thought she needed to take care of me. And that was another role she wasn't accustomed to. We're each the youngest in our families and neither of us had any experience taking care of others. Even in our marriage we split up all of our duties. Although she did the bulk of the housework, attending to my needs was not in her job description.

With grace, however, Cheryl was excited to be a caretaker, to give herself completely. I was the one who caused her need to give to be frustrating because, being self-sufficient most of my life, I couldn't allow her to take care of me. Aside from the two weeks when I was completely laid up, I was back trying to make my own meals, cart myself around and take care of my own things. Cheryl was left wondering what her role was. Should she go ahead and do everything for me or should she assume I really didn't need her and let me fend for myself?

I did need her but I didn't know how to show it. I knew I didn't need her in a service way, lying on the couch with a cold compress on my forehead. "Dear, could you get me a cool drink please?" "Honey, I think my bandage needs changing." "Cheryl, would you mind so much rubbing my temples, and while you're at it, could you plant a garden, strip and re-stain the windows, and, if you have the time, could you gut an antelope for me?"

Whether she would have or not, I didn't want to need her like that. I didn't marry to have someone do things for me. How I needed her was more subtle than how she took care of me. Cheryl made me feel complete even as she sat in despair about not being able to give me the things she thought I needed. She treated me like a human being. And human beings do all these things. Loving another person has little to do with gifts or gratifying or running errands; it has more to do with kinship, honesty and profound respect. She eased my greatest fear of cancer — losing my humanity. I was afraid of turning into some *thing*, and Cheryl wouldn't let that happen in our house.

She wasn't afraid to yell at me and that was one of the ways she kept me human. Like a mother fearing for her children's safety scolds her kids when they endanger their own being, Cheryl scolded me. Ours, I hope, was not like a mother/child relationship, but there were parallels between the emotions. I spent an entire week in chemo, remembering about six hours of it, and would then come home and fully expect the house to run as it did before I left. From her perspective, that was ridiculous. She had been a single parent, making dinners on her own, paying bills, entertaining, caring for and disciplining children as well as personal coping for the duration of my absence. My fitting in seamlessly was totally out of the question. Yet, every week, as if I were a four-year-old testing my boundaries, I did the same thing all over again.

I never fully understood Cheryl's point. Maybe it was the effects of the Attivan or a guilty need to be involved or perhaps it was that I had just experienced the equivalence of being of cryogenically frozen for the week. At any rate, from the moment I reached the house, I tried to catch up on parenting the kids. "Let me fix your hair, Dylan." "Why are you chewing gum?" "You kids go outside and give your mother a break." Wanting to be the dad I was, with my hand in household matters and feeling guilty for having left Cheryl for an entire week (again), I thought I could pick up the slack. I thought my coming home each week was going to magically lift her burden — or at least I wanted it to, but looking back I don't know what I was thinking. By commandeering the kids I was to compensate for the impotent feeling of having cancer.

That was when Cheryl would yell at me. Although yelling isn't the right term because she hardly has that kind of voice or demeanor, for her it was an explosion. She pointed out that I was in no position to assume responsibilities. Not only was I not helping by trying to jump right into the thick of our family life, but I was actively working against it. In one sense, for me to be home at all was trouble. "Don't you understand?" she pleaded with me. "Even if you did all the things you normally did, make dinners, pay bills and be the dad, in a couple weeks you're going to leave all over again. You'll abandon your jobs and I'll have to start back at square one. Then we'll fight for control all over again when you come back." I didn't understand. "As long as I'm here, why not help?" I reasoned. Cheryl held her ground. "Play with Matthew. Play cards and games with Rachel and Dylan. Be a fun uncle while you're home. You're just not in a position to be a dad. You don't even have to be Scott. Just be a boarder if that's what it takes. You're sick and your only job is to not be sick anymore."

As we fought and I kept not understanding, Cheryl's combativeness came from the most genuine sense of love I could have asked for. It was what I needed most from her. She recognized, even as I didn't want to, that our lives had changed considerably. She fought with me for my own sake so that I could focus on the strenuous battle I needed to face 24 hours a day. It was confusing, but her emotional tension grew because of both my ignorance as well as the responsibility that accompanied heading the family. By uniquely combining love and toughness we maintained our sanity.

Although she was angry when she needed to be, there were also the moments when she came to me as a precious angel. I remember two separate times when I had more of cancer than I could handle: once at home after my allograph and once toward the end of chemo. Both times I fell into depression and both times Cheryl was there. When chemo was burning me so I couldn't eat at home and it felt like it was hollowing me out, I told Cheryl I'd had enough. I told her that if God left the decision up to me whether to live or die, I would have gone with death. The words felt strange even as I said them; I didn't understand them or accept them myself. Yet Cheryl, looking at me with her tired and gentle eyes and touching me with her calming hands, understood.

But the defining moment for Cheryl and me came after the bone transplant. The complete uselessness of my leg, along with the fear that cancer would never end and a sharp pain running down my back left me one night at a new level of despair. I felt I had gone insane, as if nothing made sense to me. In tremendous pain, I couldn't remember when it started or imagine it ever ending. I forgot about my children, my wife, God, and even my own life. The only way I could express myself was by sprawling out in our living room and banging my head on our hardwood floors.

That was Cheryl's first real opportunity to take care of me. She'd spent so much time worrying whether she could do the things she was supposed to do. But all those things she was supposed to do were just for show, to make *her* feel better. On the floor, although I didn't know it, I needed her more than ever. Normally she'd have to think of the right thing to do, but in this case it was glaringly obvious and she did it without knowing she answered the call. Cheryl came to me on the floor and rubbed my body, my back, shoulders and legs — no pretensions, no plan. She didn't talk to me or try to tell me everything was all right because she knew it wasn't. Once again, her understanding was exactly what I needed. She stayed with me and relief came, not because of what she did but because she was there. There was no better explanation than that.

It was a moment neither of us will ever forget. So much was said without saying anything at all. U2 had a song about despair that reminded me of our night: "You've got to cry without weeping/ talk without speaking/ scream without raising your voice ..." We were both so vulnerable and in need of each other. Maybe we reached a higher level of communication. Maybe we were communicating the way we always should because we were both so human at that point. Maybe it was grace.

Cheryl is a poet. She wrote years before I had cancer, seemed to write volumes during, and has stuck with it unfailingly since. Like many other things, she has always doubted her poetry, but I never have. I believe she found her voice when I had cancer. There are many to choose from, but I often look to one poem in particular to remember my cancer, to remember our history and to remember Cheryl, my blessing.

(for J.H. and S.F.)

That summer there were prayers.
Prayers over people having coffee. Prayers single file
as the children left school. Prayers blooming out
the lips of tulips. Prayers under the obscenities
screamed from the couple across the street. Prayers
from the breath of dogs barking. One prayer laid
its head on my pillow when I remembered my husband
and me at the University hospital when the doctor said,
"I'm sorry Mr. Burton - you have Osteo Sarcoma."

Everywhere that summer prayers arrived in envelopes
from unknown people: from Wisconsin, Peoria, IL.,
Arkansas, a woman who had inherited money from her
grandmother. Prayers flew from the pen we used to
write bills, came in from calls from Omaha, Nebraska,
and not all the prayers had voices:

> *some were afraid*
> *some prayers kept coughing*
> *some prayers had arthritic fingers*
> *smelled of rotten apples*
> *picked the lint off our clothes*
> *Were made into salads and tossed*

before our dinner plates.
> *Rode over our pillows at night in horse-*
less carriages.
> *They had the voice of split tomatoes.*
Were painted black and
> *dropped from the sky like the juice*
from rare meat before placed on the tongue.

There were prayers that grew large black spots consuming me
faster than the cells in my husband's leg. Prayers that were larger
than life. Prayers with scales of a snake. Prayers heavy round boulders:

> *prayers taking up oxygen*
> *prayers putting my children to bed*

prayers pointing fingers and whispering

Where were the prayers for the children in Somalia,
for my father who lost his wife, for the other
cancer victims.

The prayers were pregnant with prayer babies already named
after us. Prayers fell on St. Helena's church sticking to crosses.
Prayers fought with the hymns arguing over Catholic Doctrine.
Prayers made faces at the ugly children dressed in bows and looking
like apes.

Prayers grew supple and leaned on my shoulder. Prayers built alters
of lust. Prayers taunted their celibacy.

Prayers grew into the shape of my brother, inhabited my atheistic
father. Whispered strange poems in my husband's ear, "Squeaky
little pigs with inflatable headwear..."

> Prayers dressed in high heels,
> battled with God,
> bought tickets to New Orleans and split.

Prayers mimicked my husband on crutches, not out of snottiness,
but sympathy.

Prayers flowed through IV bags filled
with Adriamyacin straight to my husband's heart

making him groggy and sleep, forgetting he hadn't
eaten for seven days.

Prayers were rolled up into Lotus Spring rolls,
the one food he could eat afterwards.

Prayers vomited out his stomach in foam smelling
of bile and the sea. Prayers ate a hole in his mother

like battery acid.

Prayers covered my children in a thick syrup,
chasing after them down the street.

Prayers wondered aloud.
Believed in the end,
didn't believe in the end.
Held onto God's leg,
wore the dress of Sainthood

and didn't want the baggage of all the other prayers.

Near the end of my chemo some blessed angels of another sort held a benefit filling the Guthrie Theater to raise money for our family. We were given a video tape of the show, and about a year after my recovery, Cheryl and I were watching it. She laughed along with the entertainers, feeling the warmth of that night. At the end of the show, Cheryl and I walked on stage to offer our overwhelmed thank you to everyone who gave so much kindness and love. Watching that part intently, she turned to me and said, "Wow! I can't believe how *bad* you looked."

I guess even grace wears off.

Baby You Can Drive My Car
(Freedom)

By the time I reached the second half of chemo, it dawned on me how much I had left to go through before I would be done. I felt like I was nearing the finish of a 100 mile race only to find that all my running, pain and sweat had only gotten me up to the starting line. Not only wasn't chemo simple but it had become surreal — as if I were living two lives. I could have sworn I spent most of my time sleeping in my dark room, yet I remember people kept coming in and interacting as I chatted, laughed and, occasionally, threw up. Maybe it was an out of body experience. I recall visitors coming in my room one after another as if they were Sicilians lined up outside seeking an audience with Don Corleone. At the same time I saw myself asleep in my bed in an empty room. If it was a dream, I wasn't aware which one was real and which wasn't.

Because of the way chemo had begun to dominate me at the hospital, I valued dearly my time at home. Things changed when I started seeing that my time at home was no longer about scurrying for work, writing, making money or being a dad and husband. My times back home were brief vacations away from cancer. I'd always imagined that when people are told they only have a short time to live, they embrace what they love and forget everything else. For weeks at a time, I was able to live like that. Released from responsibility, I lived without the burden of life.

Cheryl and I talked a lot during these respites. Not that we didn't talk before but I'd become less agenda oriented. We talked about a number of things — heparin (the blood thinning solution I injected in to clean my catheter), pills, doctors, life and death — as casually as if we were discussing a movie we'd just seen. Like Tony, I didn't pretend to have answers; I just needed to talk. But the medical talks and talks about the direction of our lives led to open discussions about the children, friends, our kind neighbors next door and a wider, happier view on life.

Now that I had accepted putting the rest of my life on hold, I spent more time with the kids. Because most of my time I was sitting on the floor or on the couch rehabilitating my leg, I was about the same height as Matthew. It was so easy to hold him, let him climb on me or sit and play with him. All I needed to do was wear my bright red hat, and he would spend half the day pawing me to reach it, taking it off and putting it back on first his head then mine. With Rachel and Dylan, I could sit at the little table Cheryl had set up in their room and watch or help them with play-doh. Sometimes I'd lay on the floor between the two downstairs bedrooms as Rachel and I rolled a car to each other along the hardwood hallway floor. Dylan and I rolled a ball between ourselves, our legs open in a V, toes touching. It was good to be a dad again.

Although I couldn't completely stop worrying, without paying attention to it or trying, I was given a new life every time I went home. It was a life with no pressure that I couldn't take for granted if I wanted to. Years after cancer, I learned that few other survivors had that luxury. A friend I had made, Jim Van Hercke, told of how he had to go for radiation treatments over his lunch hour and return to work so no one would know he had Hodgkin's disease. Although his battle occurred over 20 years ago, the fear of job security looms over so many other survivors even today. Being self-employed and having saved enough money for us to live off of for a few months, I didn't feel great stress about not working. I was graced with some fortunate blessings that were unique to my situation; not having to work was one of them.

Yet strangely, with all the gifts I had after recovering from a disabling chemo, I didn't notice one of the greatest gifts right under my own nose: I didn't need my crutches anymore. But I couldn't know it until the hospital specifically told me when. For me to understand, I needed Dr. Thompson to say something like, "At exactly 3:15 on July 14th, your leg will be strong enough to walk without crutches." I often forgot that I could determine my own rate of rehabilitation. There is no pre-determined time a person has to be on crutches just as there is no exact time a person has to wait to go swimming after a meal (though waiting a half hour is a good idea, really). After my allograph and the brutal and painful recovery, I accepted that my rehab schedule was at the mercy of others.

After the bone transplant I was given a heavy leg brace that ran the length of my leg. It had eight velcro straps and an adjustable hinge so that I could bend it to varying degrees. In the beginning I kept it locked straight, but after having a pin removed from my knee, it was set for a 30 degree bend so as to start my recovery. I was also given a Passive Motion Machine that I could strap into which bent my knee up and down. Dr. Thompson explained that the machine's purpose was to break scar tissue building up in the knee joint.

About a month had gone by before I realized I had misunderstood him once again. I thought the machine was somehow exercising the muscles in my leg, but I knew by then it wasn't. My first giveaway should have been the fact that it was a motorized device, moving my leg all on its own. I have yet to see any weight rooms in which you sit strapped idle on a moving machine and receive a complete muscular workout. If there were such places I'm sure they would be huge successes since anybody could get a full body workout as they napped. But one need only visit a local golf course to see that riding around on a motorized vehicle and perfect muscle tone don't exactly go hand in hand.

In spite of my ignorance, I hooked into that contraption four hours a day, content with my schedule. The only real drawback to the machine was, being an older model, it was terribly loud — almost too loud to carry on a conversation. As I sat on the couch, strapped in, staring out the window, I would feel as if I were on the tarmac at O'Hare airport during departure time. When Cheryl came in to ask me if I wanted a salad or something, it was like watching TV with the volume down.

Since my machine was made of fused metal with a crude motor and weighed a ton, I estimated that it was manufactured sometime in the late 1800s from leftover railroad ties and excess freight. Perhaps it was created by the same guy who invented the hard hospital mattresses and mixed chemo. Emotionally, I wanted to get away from that machine, unstrap myself and run. But logically, and assuming I wouldn't be off crutches for a year, I was satisfied with my slow progress. So the combination of contentedness, ignorance and the mind-numbing noise worked to my advantage, helping me not be impatient, and to work hard for full use of my leg.

Somewhere along the line, I think early July, my rehabilitation started to feel a little too easy. About the same time I realized the machine wasn't exercising my leg, I began to ask questions. "All I need to do is sit here and this machine will rehabilitate my leg?" I wondered. "There must be something else. Maybe I'm ready for the next step." As fate would have it, my questions were answered before I even had time to ask another.

At my next checkup, between chemo three and four, before I could even ask what the next step was, Dr. Thompson pulled out of a box a brand new, lighter, less restrictive leg brace. It was made of a maroon, velvety material with spongy stuff on the inside. And it only had two straps! As Dr. Thompson held it, I looked at the brace like King Arthur gazing on the Holy Grail. It was so small, so simple — a new world. "You mean," I was thinking, like a kid getting a car for graduation, "that's for *me*?" Since I was still on crutches, having Dr. Thompson bring out that wonderful new piece of equipment showed how far off I was with my un-ambitious schedule. I was hoping for a faster, quieter machine. Eager, but not wanting to jump to conclusions, I let him show how the brace worked and a physical therapist came in to go over some of the do's and don'ts of the apparatus. Only then, as Cheryl and I were about to leave, did I say to him, "So does this mean I can walk without crutches now?" Dr. Thompson is such a reserved and polite man but even he must've been thinking, "Well, *Duh!*"

That was the first step, my first glimpse at how rapidly life would change with more mobility. Almost immediately I re-aligned my views on physical recovery. Whereas once I was sitting on the couch, hooked up to the passive motion machine, thinking how great it was I that could make meals and watch TV, with the new brace I began thinking things like, "I wonder if I can jog with this thing?" I started remembering all the things I used to be able to do. While I walked around like Bambi on newborn legs and imagined all that lay ahead of me, time seemed to fly by as I walked stronger, straighter, and more confidently every day.

I had reached the point where I could walk with hardly a limp when it hit me. There I was in my living room thinking normal, everyday thoughts — "I wonder what the kids are up to today?" "Where did I put that crossword puzzle?" "Man! Those Monkees were a great band!" — when out of nowhere it popped into my head: "Hey, I can drive the car! I can drive! I can walk outside, swing the door open, put the key in the ignition, turn it and tool around wherever I want." Of my entire recovery, that was the most glorious, freeing and earth shattering revelation. It took about three weeks longer than it should have and felt like one of those discoveries that you wish you could have back, like a first date or missing a tax deduction. But "better late than never" could not have been a more apt cliché.

A couple of years earlier, driving would have seemed like the simplest, most mundane job, something anyone over the age of 16 would have taken for granted. But having it taken away and then given back to me put driving at the top of my growing list of freedoms. After the cadaverous allograph and nine hours of surgery, it was a freedom to simply get up in bed. Other freedoms were using the wheelchair, crutching out into the hallway and even using the bathroom by myself. Each step I took, each word I spoke, the little jokes I made to the staff, every laugh expressed was exercising my freedom. When all else failed, I had those laughs and conversations to tell me what life truly meant. But driving was a different kind of freedom — my first physical one. I wasn't juggling or back on stage, but now I felt they were possible. Fittingly, driving was the first freedom that put me on the road to getting there.

Driving also had a special place in my heart. Since the day I got my learner's permit — even before that, in the high school auto simulator — I loved driving. Perhaps it was the sense of control or the feeling of going somewhere or maybe it was because I could do it alone, but driving put me at ease. My dad told me after I got my permit that I was going to get sick of it awfully soon, but that has yet to happen. Half of my days are spent in the car and it's still one of my favorite places to be. Even when I was traveling 20,000 miles a year doing college shows, the drive was often the most enjoyable part of the trip. Regardless of the reason — going on long trips with my family, short rides to the post office, driving my brother around from L.A. — I never tired of it.

When I was in high school, I used to take Jack's metallic blue

Pinto and drive slowly through the streets of Edina, an upscale suburb of Minneapolis. I would put some music on the radio, soak up the view and just let thoughts drift across my mind. My drives were similar to the long walks some people enjoy: They afforded a lazy kind of soul searching. Occasionally I'd stop the car to look at a nice house or beautiful park or even stare at the sky; then I'd mosey on again like a stranger passing through town. Never having a time limit or anywhere to go, I kept driving until I thought of something else to do or until an Edina resident called the police because a car of overwhelming tackiness was roaming their city limits.

The funny part of my driving epiphany was that I didn't act on it right away. Usually when I get an idea, I do it without consulting others. But I was so excited that the first thing I did was tell Cheryl. "I bet I can drive," I told her while showing how much I could bend my leg. "I bet I can drive," I said all over again because she didn't jump up and down with glee saying, "Oh good, Scott, I'm so excited for you" the first time. It made sense that she was leery. The last thing you want to hear from a person who has limited mobility in his leg and who's been taking near fatal drugs on a monthly basis is, "Hey, whaddya say we pile all the kids in the car and see if I can control the darn thing." She wanted to be happy for me and wanted me to have something I could revel in, but, with my history in the hospital and my leg not completely healed, she had a hard time consenting.

But that didn't stop me. After the first hour of waiting expect-antly for Cheryl to let me get behind the wheel , I figured an immediate agree-ment wasn't going to come. So as she deliberated, I sat in the parked car practicing moving my foot from the gas pedal to the brake. Eventually, with her reluctant approval, I drove leisurely once again and with great pride. I drove through town with the wide-eyed gawkiness of Jethro Bodine when the Clampetts reached Beverly Hills. It was almost a dream. Only two months from a limb-saving operation and faced with death, I was back behind the wheel of a small car going absolutely nowhere.

It was while driving that I imagined what would be my next step. I thought of traveling, of sports and again envisioned myself performing. But the next freedom I embraced was the simple, joyful freedom I craved all along — juggling once more. I hadn't picked up my props since diagnosis. Like getting off crutches, I didn't expect to juggle for another year or so. But while driving I passed a familiar lake, and looking towards the shore I imagined myself with thick blonde hair, with a larger and stronger wrestler's body and weathered juggler's hands, tossing clubs to the amusement of people passing by.

Juggling was so ingrained in who I was that it was the physical expression of all my other freedoms. At the time I didn't know what it represented, I just wanted to do it. I'd been waiting a long time, almost lulling myself into not caring about it anymore. But the moment came in spite of myself. I was going to juggle.

As fate would have it, my best juggling partner and good friend Bryan Wendling was in town from Kansas City at the same time I had my revelation. Bryan is simply one of the best jugglers in the country. We juggled together every chance we got, which wasn't often; because we lived in different states and because of my cancer diagnosis, we hadn't passed clubs in almost a year. Also, the growing friendship between our two families — Cheryl and Bryan's wife Fabi had become close — meant we no longer had to juggle all the time. But given this golden opportunity, knowing I could juggle and knowing he was nearby, I called him. "Hey, Bob," I said (long ago Bryan used to perform under the name "Bob the Incredible Juggler" and I still use both names interchangeably like a bilinguist), "I think I can juggle. Care to head on down to the lakes with me?" In Minneapolis, because the weather is favorable for just over four or five weeks out of the year, when it's nice out that's where jugglers go. Bryan is pretty good at hiding any discomfort, so if he thought it was a stupid idea, I didn't notice. So we met at Lake of the Isles. I, of course, drove.

Out on a glade overlooking the lake, I was worked my body like an emancipation. I passed clubs around my back, through my legs and felt my muscles moving in every direction. Just manipulating those clubs, twirling and catching them was enough to complete my life. Nobody knew how it felt, not even Bryan, and he was there. But I knew. It was the feeling that the best freedom of all is being alive and everything else is a bonus. My greatest fear, that I would lose my humanity, left me that day.

I felt so good, so normal that I almost felt cured. The pessimist in me was waiting for something to go wrong: an assassination attempt, a nuclear holocaust, a total eclipse, something to take that wonderful feeling away. But even if it were taken away, I had already tasted it. Hanging out with Bryan and watching him juggle was familiar, but the feelings that accompanied it took me to a whole new world. With just a little more magic, it would have been like the scene when Dorothy landed in Oz. I was Dorothy, standing by the lake with Bryan and my prop bag, while the enigmatic pink crystal bubble floated over the trees of the island, glided gently above the lake and alighted in front of me. In the background, Munchkins watched as the bubble transformed into a beautiful fairy. And with a wide, bright smile that I normally would think was phony, the beautiful woman spoke in her high, squeaky, fair witch's voice: "Are you a good juggler or a bad juggler?"

"Well, I really don't want to commit on that right now. I haven't done it for quite some time you know."

"Why, you silly boy. You've had the power to juggle all along."

"I have?"

"Why yes. All you need to do is knock your juggling clubs together three times and say 'I have some free time, I have some free time.'" Like Dorothy, I smiled knowingly. "Yes. Yes, I see now. I'm ready. I'm ready to juggle again." The Munchkins tittered from behind a bush. But as I stood before the lake and the open sky, I knew I didn't need the magic of Oz. I had a wonderful reality. And, unlike my time in chemo, there was no disputing it *was* reality. The laughter wasn't Munchkins, only some little kids gawking — but I could have sworn one of them had a beard.

The magic was feeling young and strong again, forgetting I was bald and 20 pounds lighter. Although I felt young and eternal, I could only imagine what it looked like to other people. Seeing jugglers at the lake is enough to turn a person's head to begin with. Seeing a shiny-white, stick-like person in the midst of chemotherapy juggling at the lake is another matter altogether. What went through those peoples' minds? I could just imagine the elderly ladies with wealthy husbands and good pensions, wearing their almost-matching exercise suits and walking their small, nondescript, short-haired dogs around the lake.

"Say, Bev, is that a totally hairless young man with a leg brace and skin just a tad whiter than school paste juggling over there by the geese?"

"Why yes, Gladys, I do believe it is."

"Isn't that illegal here?"

"I'm not sure. We *are* pretty progressive in this state you know."

I suppose there was some curiosity, probably some well-good-for-him attitudes. I'm sure there was some fear looking at me. But probably the most common reaction of those who saw me was pity since that was what I usually got. I was at the point in my treatment where I could have stood on a street corner with a sign around my neck that said "Pity me" and made a substantial living. But the feelings I had were so good I could ignore the pity. Bob and I were *juggling*.

We practiced our individual routines and, while my strength was not what it used to be, I could do nearly all of my old tricks: spins, twists, juggling through my legs and all around my body. It was hard but we rekindled the old routine that won us a national juggling championship way back in 1983, doing spins and tricks that I never thought I would do again. We passed six, seven and eight clubs while doing tricks. We passed eight clubs between us over our heads while standing back to back, and though it was difficult for my tired body, we passed nine clubs. There was one revelation I probably never would have experienced without having cancer. Watching the clubs fly and feeling my muscles tire, it occurred to me, "I *get* to do this. I *get* to be here right now! I *get* to tell my story." Breathing hard and with sweat running down my temples, I finished my routine with a spin: In more ways than one, I got it.

It was as if doors opened up from then on. Some agents called me about work, friends were organizing the benefit at the Guthrie, and I was asked to write a script for the TV show "Roseanne." As the doors began to swing open freely, I was like a 5 year-old with a dollar at the candy store. Maybe I was a little too cocky. After driving downtown to pick up my mail, I cruised down the main drag, curving down by the Basilica of St. Mary's, heading toward Uptown all the while thinking, "I *could* be going to Kinko's right now. If I really wanted to mail a letter, I could. Maybe I'll just drive over to Taco Bell, walk right in, without crutches, and order some food. I just might."

Ironically, as it was a metaphoric door that allowed me to be free, it was an actual door that became my undoing. While driving and thinking of errands to do, I decided to visit the warehouse space in North Minneapolis where I had practiced for the past ten years, the place where I had honed all my juggling skills. I had worked harder than anywhere else I've worked in my life. I spent two to three hours a day juggling while I blasted a boombox so loud it could be heard on the floor above the thick concrete ceilings. Each day after working out, repetitively learning the tricks that Bob and I did at Lake of the Isles, I could wring out my shirt and drain nearly a half a glass of sweat out of it.

I wasn't going back to juggle but to just stand in the space, reconnect myself with my past and my passion. There was a dart board there so I thought I'd throw for a while or just sit on the couch and soak in the air. Maybe I'd even practice again. Walking up to the door — a typical, office-building, heavy plate glass door — I stepped my left leg in and something on the side of the door hooked my shirt on the left shoulder, twisting me halfway around. I then heard the most sickening crack. Knowing the glass on the door hadn't broken, I had no doubt as to what had happened. I didn't need any special training to know what that jerking twist and awful cracking sound could have been. I had broken my leg.

Even though my instinct told me what had happened, my brain hadn't caught up. I put into use the only medical advice I received during five years on the Roosevelt High School wrestling team: walk it off. If I put some weight on my leg by walking on it, the pain might go away. Barely able to walk, I went into the warehouse, limped down the stairs and visited my juggling space anyway. Darts were out of the question. Even sitting down on the couch wasn't appealing anymore. My brain finally caught up with the rest of my body and said I'd better get back home and call Dr. Thompson.

Driving home I was angry with myself, wondering what the heck I was thinking. Did I have to push myself so hard? Why did I have to do everything in one day? I wanted that moment back again so badly. It was like trying to retrieve a letter I didn't mean to drop in the mailbox or closing the locked door of my car knowing the keys were in there. I just wanted to jump back. I wanted there to have been a large sign on the door that said, "Hey Scott, watch out! Tuck your shirt in — this door's a killer."

The clinic got me in right away and Dr. Thompson confirmed what my instincts had already told me. The juncture inside my thigh where the new allograph bone was grafted to my femur twisted itself so that the bones were no longer in union. That meant I not only had to go back on crutches but needed another operation to re-graft the bones. Since the same bone would be used, the good news was I wouldn't need another nine hour allograph. But Dr. Thompson would have to shave some bone from my hip to lay down where the bones met to help the my two femurs grow together again. And, because the bone graft probably wouldn't take while I was still on chemotherapy, I would have to wait for healing. That meant I would be on crutches for the rest of my treatments.

That break took a lot of wind out of my sails. When I juggled at the lake, I was so careful that nothing would go wrong — checking the position of the sun for an eclipse, making sure there was no lone gunman on a grassy knoll — that I couldn't imagine my freedom being taken away by a simple door. To this day I think to myself, "Open the door *fully* now." I was worried that the bad news ball might start rolling again. *They were going to put me back on Methotrexate. I'd get lackluster and complacent about my rehabilitation again. The cancer would come back.*

But those worries didn't consume me. My taste of complete freedom had given me a new knowledge. In spite of the break and the ensuing depression, I had seen the place where I wanted to be again, at the lake juggling or on stage doing a show. I knew the possibilities and I knew they were within my reach.

"Put Me In Coach, I'm Ready To Play... Uh, What Game Is This?"

By the fourth treatment, chemo had become routine. Weathering the storm for three and a half months had made all that had happened and was yet to happen no longer feel out of the ordinary. Going to the hospital was like going to Rachel's weekly basketball games. Except for how I looked and that it came up in nearly every conversation, I would have forgotten I *had* cancer. All the miracles of medicine, limb saving operations and killing my body to let it live again had blended into the same let's-get-it-over-with experience.

The doctors talked to me every week and I almost stopped listening. "Mr. Burton, we are working, even now, on new and more effective chemos for your cancer." "Uh, huh," I'd say. "Hey, you know what!? I think I'm double-jointed!"

Chemotherapy, which is almost as experimental today as applying leeches used to be, had become the same old thing. Maybe that was how it had to be. Every level of life, no matter how incredible, must have some kind of complacency factor built into it. If we remained fascinated at every amazing aspect of life, we'd still be staring at our hands, wiggling our fingers and picking stuff up saying, "This is *so* cool. These little things at the end of my hands do whatever I want them to!"

I compared my own numbing repetition to that of a professional football player's life. Every single week those guys take part in a perception-altering experience. For football players, their routine is millions of fans getting together and screaming in their ears, revering them as gods in a stadium where the energy is at a fever pitch for two solid hours. Their emotional intensity reaches near life and death levels every week. I would think each moment for those guys would be unique and memorable. Yet I'm sure some of those guys sum up their larger-than-life jobs with, "Well, I run into people, they fall down, then they get up." The altering of my existence was caused by the drugs, living in a hospital and the dwindling of my body. My struggle for existence revolved around every chemo, yet I could sum up my death-defying job with, "Well, I go into the hospital, get dreadfully sick, then I throw up." The other difference was they got paid ungodly sums of money for their efforts, while I was *paying* ungodly sums of money. (Actually I would be amazed if any professional football players *didn't* perceive their lives as just one long game. Especially considering that taking repeated blows to the head is part of their job description.)

The memories of the last half of chemo floated through my mind like a disorganized photo album. When I remembered a visit, a new medicine or a thought, it was hard to know if it was a recent memory, a memory of that week, the week before or third grade. Sometimes I couldn't even be sure if I was recollecting my own experience or someone else's. It was no wonder the weeks blended together: Not only had I endured the repetitive grind of chemo, but I had also ingested enough drugs to drop a musk ox.

I couldn't always remember exactly *when*, but I often remembered *what* happened. I submitted a script to "Seinfeld" during that time (which they never returned because, in my loopy state, I'd forgotten to include my address or phone number). I remember talking about comedy with my nurse for over an hour. I remember conversations with roommates, family and friends. I also remember throwing up after eating at Taco Bell and noting how both versions of the meal looked eerily similar. But while my memories flew around me like an impossible juggling trick, the benefit of forgetting so much was I hardly paid attention to my life passing by.

For the most part, I didn't mind not having full control of my memory. But I wondered what made one memory stick out in my mind while another could be forgotten. For example, I didn't remember leaving Masonic 3 and walking to the nearby Lotus restaurant, pulling along my IV stand, yet Cheryl told me I did. But I remembered sitting outside near the front sidewalk of the hospital, IV stand, crutches and all. I had hobbled out the doors, through the gang of defiant smokers-on-chemo, then out to a recessed area of the front sidewalk that was made into a long bench. I propped my leg up along the bench, watched the college kids go by, and daydreamed. I sang songs to myself, pretended I knew some of the students and thought of comedy bits. *That* I remember — not walking with anyone else, not going to the restaurant, not wandering the halls of the cancer ward.

I think the reason I remembered being on the bench was because, while I was there, I so badly wanted to have a concept of time. That bench was the one place where I felt I had control of myself. I was alone, it was quiet and I didn't have to explain myself to anyone — including me. In my room the air was stifling and the chemo smell was all around me. At home with Cheryl and the kids, I was free but I was still Dad, a husband — I was still Scott. On the bench, I was just a guy living the life God had breathed into me, with no plan. It was a combination of the life without responsibility I had at home and the comfort of not fearing cancer.

But even when I thought I had control, it seemed as if time had stopped when I was out there. I was on the bench, feeling the breeze and the sun like I was tanning on a beach in California. My mind took in memories like a deep breath, but by the time I grew tired and headed back in, it felt as if only half an hour had passed. I was angry because I wished I were stronger and could stay there to eat up more chemo time. But after getting to my room, I'd see that well over an hour, sometimes more than two, had passed. It was like getting upset about not being able to find my glasses, then after a couple of hours, realizing they were on my head all along.

Even though it was the best place to be while in chemo, I didn't go outside much. It was weird, almost as if the power of Attivan helped me to forget that I was even *allowed* to go outside. My waking thoughts were often only a recognition of where I was. I woke up sporadically throughout each day thinking, "What am I doing here? Why do I feel so spacey? Oh right, I'm in chemo. I wonder what's on TV." There were times when, without noticing, I found myself outside thinking, "Hey, look, I'm outside!" But while in my bed, I never remembered thinking, "Hey, I *should* go outside."

My inability to remember what I'd done or why I'd done it was exactly why Cheryl was nervous every time I left my room. Once she called my room and there was no answer. She called the station to ask where I was, thinking I was getting a test, or out with someone on a visit, but the nurses said they didn't know where I'd gone. For Cheryl, that was as nerve-racking as losing a child in a crowded department store. I was out on the street and it wasn't like she could have me paged. There were only a limited number of places I could have gone, so I had to at least be in the vicinity. But that offered little consolation to Cheryl considering my state of mind. The nurses had no idea where I was. Cheryl had no idea where I was and, due to how she had seen the chemo drugs affect me, she also assumed I had no idea where I was either.

She called sometime later and that time I answered. "Where were you?"

"I've been here all day, Hon."

"I just called an hour ago and no one knew where you were."

"Oh. Maybe I was outside."

"You just said you were in your room all day."

"Um, I probably was. Sometimes I go outside though."

"I don't want you leaving anymore. Don't go out unless you go with somebody."

"I don't know. It's not like I have no idea what I'm doing," I said, having had no idea what I'd been doing. But I was trying to comfort her, so I assured her, "It's not like I'm walking out to the nurses station with a bottle of liquor and a bus pass saying, 'I'll be back around five or so.' But with my history in chemo, I was the last person she was going to take advice from. Cheryl had her own images of what could happen to me: wandering in on a class at the University or getting mugged or walking away and not knowing the way back to the hospital. Little did she know I was enjoying myself on the bench out front passing time and wishing I had guts to heckle the passing medical students; "Man, this new hands-on pre-med final is a killer!" Because of that episode Cheryl asked the nurses not to let me walk off the floor without accompaniment.

One other consistent memory was tangling with the terribly sweet lunch lady who came into my room each day and asked whether or not I was going to eat. I never caught (or remembered) her name, so I'll call her Doreen. She was a petite woman with a friendly smile and snowy gray hair — completely unlike any of the lunch ladies I remember from high school, some of whom are now working as the professional football players I'd mentioned. Even though I hadn't had a bite all week, Doreen, that kind woman, would enter my room acting as if I hadn't refused food the entire week before. She would peek her head around the corner and step in like a child waking her parents at 6 a.m. on a Saturday and ask, "Would you like a tray today?" "Oh, I don't think so," I'd say. I hated turning her down and yet was a little resentful that she just kept coming like a well-meaning stalker. Doreen's was a caring perseverance but I thought that, by the fourth chemo, she would have just given up. She knew I didn't want to eat, but that woman tried everything.

"Would you like a tray today?"

"No, thank you."

"How about a shake? A lot of patients who can't eat have these high calorie shakes. A lot of nutrients. Yum."

"I don't think so."

"Can you eat some fruit?"

"I'd love to, but no."

Not only did I not want to eat, I didn't even want to think about eating. But I couldn't escape it. The moment petite Doreen and her cart reached the floor, that suffocating cafeteria smell interacted with the horrible hospital stench and created a brand new nauseating odor that floated through the halls like some kind of poison gas on "Star Trek." Ironically, the smell of food was a bad memory even though, besides the hoagie and the peach, I didn't eat any food throughout chemo. It wasn't just that I couldn't get the food down, but, considering the sheer volume of how much I was throwing up, I didn't think of it as eating so much as re-loading. I felt bad turning her down, but because she kept coming, I almost wanted to shout when the odor reached me, "Scott's not in this room. He had an appointment to go to. This is Steve and I've already eaten."

Although the smell of the food, the smell at the elevators and the drab hospital floors remain memories to this day, I seem to have forgotten at least half of my visits. I remember people being there, and I remember select conversations, but I don't remember many of them. And I wish I did because it was profoundly encouraging that friends did come. Since I didn't remember, they had to explain later, "Oh yeah, I was there. You seemed great. You talked, joked around and seemed really lucid." I could only reply, "You *visited* me?"

The first time it happened was when Bryan and Fabi came up from Kansas City. Fabi, a beautiful and bright-eyed woman from Ecuador, with thick and long curled black hair, could hardly believe me. Always ready for a laugh, she thought I was joking and maintained that she and Bryan had visited earlier, recounting how good I appeared. Being the first time anyone said something like that, it blew my mind. Fabi went into detail of what we talked about and seemed so assured of her presence that there was nothing I could say. Eventually I conceded and said, "Well, I'm sure glad you came." But I still wasn't convinced.

Bill Arnold, one of my best friends, not only visited but also had driven me to the hospital for a couple of my operations. Bill is an entertainer too, and a top-notch one at that. We met at a comedy club called the Rib Tickler where we both worked regularly, he as a comic/magician. Sharing a passion for faith and a slightly cynical sense of humor, Billy and I became fast friends. Before my cancer episode, we met regularly for breakfast, swapping stories about our latest gigs and the agents in town who booked us into bizarre shows or endlessly tried to whittle down our prices. They were always inside jokes because the average layperson doesn't know that the natural enemy of the entertainer is the entertainer's agent ("Mutual of Omaha's Wild Kingdom" did a show on that once). Billy and I would often fret over the uncertainty of our careers and then, to break up the mood, he'd tell me his latest agent story:

"Say, Bill, I have this client, a major corporation," the agent begins. "I think this could be some excellent exposure for you, and I know your show would be a perfect fit for their local fund-raiser. Uh, by the way, would you by any chance own your own gorilla costume?"

Then I would tell mine:

"Hi, Scott. I've got a client that represents a business that doesn't have a lot of money, but they're really interested in having you. They think your magic act is a natural tie-in to their product."

"Uh, yeah, that sounds great but I don't do magic. I'm a juggler."

"Oh? Is there a difference?"

"Um, no. Not in the grand scheme of things. I guess not."

"Great. You'll be the opening act for the headliner. Have you ever worked with Bobo before?"

"I don't think so."

"Well, just don't mess around with his exploding shoes. They're pretty touchy."

Billy said that at the hospital we talked about the same things. It was during one breakfast after chemo that he told me that I had my vomiting down to a perfect science and was able to give a new twist to our agent stories. He explained that once when he visited, I sat in my bed with my spit pan in front of me. I then did my impression of an entertainer visiting his agent. "You want to pay me how much?" I asked indignantly. Then I proceeded to woof my guts out into the pan. When he told me that story, Billy and I overlooked the grossness of the joke and laughed out loud like we used to. Then I stopped, thought about it and said, "You *visited* me?"

There were several other people who visited that I honestly don't remember having been there. I hope that doesn't mean their visits had any less impact or that I was any less thankful for their concern. Their graciousness, I'm certain, has been noted somewhere, by God or, most importantly, in their own hearts. My inability to acknowledge them not only left my friends uncertain, but it also opened the door for other less noble people to take advantage of my situation by saying they had visited. Luckily that didn't happen. Not once did I receive a letter saying, "Thanks for switching back to AT&T. It was nice meeting you." Nor did anyone call saying, "Hi, Scott! Glad to have you on the Amway team."

Like most survivors, I had more people concerned for my well being than I could have known. For every person who visited there were five others who didn't, but who still did what they could. They called, they cooked us dinners, they sent us cards, letters and even money in the mail. The mother of a local comic friend had her prayer group praying for me and because I've worked nationally, people were praying for me all over the country. It was a blessed network.

One of the jugglers I used to share practice space with visited my home, serving as an envoy for the other jugglers in town. Although Jons came by to get a check or give me a check for our rehearsal space, he was also looking in on me. "All the guys are wondering how you're doing," he said. "What should I tell them?" Maybe I was trying to get back for all the down time I had in the hospital at the mercy of the staff, maybe I didn't realize how genuinely concerned they were, or maybe I was just being the same rebellious juggler I'd always been, but I said to him, "If they ask how I'm doing again, just look down at the ground, shake your head just a bit and say, 'It doesn't look good.'" Jons has a wry sense of humor, so he laughed a little and then said, "That'll work."

It was funny but I honestly didn't think he'd tell them. It was meant to be one of those tasteless jokes you don't tell others but share in confidence with those you trust. But it became a cruel joke when he did tell. It's possible that, knowing my kind of humor and hearing "Scott told me to tell you, 'It doesn't look good,'" some of the jugglers might have concluded that my spirits were intact. But some, I'm sure, didn't. The hospital, chemo and cancer had become so commonplace for me, I didn't take into consideration that my trials weren't commonplace for others.

A few months later I got my payback for my unfortunate use of comedy. Another juggler friend, Jeff Mason, who was in the midst of touring Europe while I was in treatment, finally reached me by phone a few months after chemo was over. "I'm really glad to hear your voice. I didn't know if I should believe it because the juggler's grapevine is pretty suspect, but I'd heard that you, uh … ." He couldn't quite finish the sentence. "Passed on," I filled in. "Yeah," he said. "So unless this is a really cool answering machine, I'm guessing they were wrong." I laughed and assured him all was well. It was like the game Telephone we played as children where one kid starts with a phrase, whispers it to the kid next to him and so on until the last child says the phrase out loud and it's not even close to the original. The rumor of my death was different from the kid's game in that ours was played on a worldwide scale and I was the one who unintentionally started the awful news.

I felt sorry that Jeff had to be concerned about my dying, but it did give me the unique opportunity to share a quotation from Mark Twain: "The rumors of my death have been greatly exaggerated."

Tears

Maybe the jokes had gotten a little out of hand. With real concern a friend confided that he thought I'd died, and I laughed out loud and told him I started the rumor. When other survivors recounted their cancer, their most common phrases were, "I cried and cried" or "I'd never cried so much in my life." For me, although having cancer was certainly no laugh riot, I laughed infinitely more than I cried. As a matter of fact, after knowing I had cancer, I was moody, whiney and made sarcastic remarks, but I didn't cry once.

My not crying wasn't a conscious effort. I wasn't walking around in floppy shoes and a clown suit with a big smile, waving my hands at people saying, "I have cancer and I'm not crying — I'm *laughing*!" Laughter was just my best form of expression. As I learned in my teenage years, I joked as a defense mechanism: I joked when I was afraid, but also when angry, happy, hungry and full. But laughing through pain, for me, is the yin and yang, the Alpha and the Omega, the vital thread that wove through every fabric of my life. But thinking I still had shades of denial in my life, Cheryl worried that I was setting myself up for a big fall. So even I wondered, "Was I embracing laughter and denying the other side? Was I forgetting about the yin and the Alpha?" I wanted to laugh but I didn't want to only be an empty joker, an ignorant fool. I wanted my experience to have depth.

Between Cheryl and me it had gotten to be little more than a joke, but at the time I may well have been in denial. Having seen friends and loved ones break down, it's a possible explanation as to why I didn't do the same. What bothered me about the notion of being in denial was I couldn't bear the thought that my own emotions were hidden so deeply that humor had become a guard from pain instead of an expression of life. If tears were buried in me I wanted to mine them. If I was hiding something I wanted to find it. But if there was something hidden, if I was the one who was hiding, I had no idea where to find me.

I found the answer in the very place Cheryl thought I began my denial, my youth. I don't often relate detailed stories of my childhood. They are stories that linger and will always stay with me, but not until something happens to trigger the memory do I think much about them. Cheryl often noted that, when she asked me about my childhood, I usually replied, "I don't remember all that much about it. I spent a lot of time alone, but it was pretty okay." She may have been right in making it, even though I didn't see the connection between my childhood and lack of emotion and joking. It wasn't that my childhood robbed me of my emotions as much as, when asked about the most formative and emotion-filled years of my life, I would say with little emotion, "They were all right."

My childhood was the most turbulent, uncertain and confusing time of my life, but I loved it anyway. I loved it because every moment was a challenge trying to figure out who I was. But, in doing so, every mask I tried on — the hard guy, the funny guy, the cool guy — felt awkward and untrue, so I ended each day at home unsure as to what life was. The only times I felt like I wasn't wearing a mask was when I was crying, and I did that a lot.

My first tears were not the rewarding kind. I was only five or six and crying was usually a response to teasing. I was the youngest of six kids and, while my parents were were easy on me because I was their last, my brothers and sisters harassed me double time. In truth we all harassed each other, but being the youngest, I received the trickle-down abuse from the older kids. Arlene would have a bad day so she'd lay into Debby for getting into her stuff; Debby would see Dave and mock his new haircut; Dave punches Jack for telling on him three weeks ago; Jack assumes the spirit of Godzilla and decimates Rose's "Midge and Friends" collection; Rose sees me and says I'm a crybaby who wets my pants. That would reduce me immediately to tears, and I would scream incoherent nonsense at her while running away, covering my ears. As I ran into each sibling from Arlene to Rose, I'd catch residual flack because I was the easiest target. Being left without a satisfying release to rage against, I'd find the dog and tell him that I think he's stupid.

It took nothing to start me bawling at that age. In some ways, I enjoyed the release of tears and the freedom to rage, but it was a child's cry, not the cathartic, fulfilling release of an adult. I cried back then for the same reason a dog barks. As a kid, crying and screaming were the only ways I knew to express myself. I didn't have the intellect or the communication skills to say, "You know, you're just calling me those names out of misplaced anger from losing that snowball fight earlier." The primal rage of tears and screaming got the point across much better. It was unproductive but the best I had to offer at the time.

As an example of how easily I cried, all my brothers or sisters had to say to set me off were two simple words: Nancy Doss. Nancy Doss was a cute little blonde girl with a ready smile whom I met at school. After playing on the front steps of her house one day, I made the mistake of telling my family of the nice time we had. "Scottie's got a girlfriend. Scottie's got a girlfriend," they taunted. "Nancy Do-oss, Nancy Do-oss." I felt as if I'd set myself up. "I don't even like her," I lied. "She's not my friend. Shaaaad-uuup," I screamed as they chased me down.

If I'd heard Nancy Doss' name spoken normally, such as in polite dinner conversation, it would have had no affect on me. But make the name bi-syllabic and say it twice, adding a mocking tone, and I would cringe like Quazimodo in the bell tower, tears pouring out of my face as I shrieked back, "Shaaaad-uuup." When riled as I was, it was proper etiquette to mutate *shut up* into that elongated interpretive version of the phrase. From my lips "shaad-uuup" meant everything from, "Leave me alone, haven't I suffered enough?" to "I don't ever want to hear that again" to "I have no choice but to take this rolling pin from the drawer and punish your shins." Occasionally I was able to wrap all possible meanings into one wretchedly annoying screech. I was taunted with other typical childhood teasing, most notably "Scotty Potty" and "Pot-head." (Ah yes, we were a clever lot.) But for some reason the Nancy Doss teasing cut me the deepest.

I grew out of the Nancy Doss phase by age ten or so, but I'd found new reasons to cry and cut loose into furious rages. Name-calling didn't affect me as much, but I started reacting to the slightest comment or criticism as an attack on my personhood. When Rose and Jack were playing cowboys, using the sawed off wooden barstools in our basement as horses, and they told me I couldn't play, I ranted and yelled like Jesse Helms at a Young Communist's Convention. My screams were more poignant, my tears more personal, my anger more venomous and I was more aware of why I was crying. Yet I understod it even less.

At that age my volitility was almost comical. Less bothered by the Nancy Doss teasing, I was looking for newer and more creative ways of feeling victimized. Once I was home alone with Jack. Although Jack has grown to be one of the most important and influential people in my life, back then we had the typical antagonistic big brother/little brother relationship. That day, as I was preparing a bath, Jack remarked on how much water I used to take one. It was a revelation for him as he went to the kitchen, filled a gallon milk carton with water and dumped it into the plugged bathtub. It hardly covered the bottom of the tub. "Look at this," he said incredulously, "Look how much water you use when you take a bath. I'll bet you use over ten gallons."

"What do you mean *me*?!" I shrieked with all the emotional stability of a hormonally unbalanced teen-aged girl. I broke down crying, "Why is it always *me*?! You know *you're* not so perfect. Why can't you leave me alone? I hate you!"

Looking back, that is the favorite irrational tirade of my life. I think about that moment and laugh. Perhaps other things had gone on and I was already at the emotional boiling point just waiting for something to give. Maybe I was on edge for days, weeks or just the past hour, but all it took was the most harmless observation for me to explode. Jack must have watched in shock, thinking, "Whoa! Perhaps a cup less suger on the Cap'n Crunch would be a good move."

It was that kind of emotion and sensitivity that was missing during my cancer. That was what Cheryl and the rest of my family were looking for. If I still had that kind of emotional bloodletting, maybe people would have felt closer to me throughout my experience, or that they could do something to help. But except for the times when I could do nothing but give up, I expressed myself by saying, "Man, I'm getting tired of all this" or else by making fun of my doctor. But who knows? If I still carried the emotional baggage of my youth, maybe I would have been too touchy to be around.

The most meaningful tears, perhaps of my whole life, were defined during my teen years. That was the first time that not only was I aware of my crying, but I knew why I was doing it. By the time I left Ericsson Elementary, I was one of the big shots in sixth grade. Although I wasn't especially good at anything except schoolwork, and I'd just started wrestling, I wore a tough guy bravado that got me a little respect. But I still didn't have any consistent friendships except a couple kids who lived in the neighborhood. Once we all moved on to a bigger school, the few pals I had at Ericsson saw they could find better and more interesting friends than me. They ventured eagerly in search of new influences, tougher attitudes and cooler swear words. Staring down the halls of Nokomis Junior high with wide-eyed excitement, they surveyed their new land. "Look at all these rooms and stand-up lockers — no cloak room. We need a special pass just to walk out into the hall. Look there! Kids my own age walking into the bathroom and *smoking*." So on the first day of school, like an early American Indian completing his rite of passage, they took a deep breath and said, "Today I am an adult."

When I looked down the same hallways, I felt more like a child than I did in elementary school. I had lost all of my old friends and was too intimidated to make new ones. I was waiting for a popular but understanding veteran student to take me under his wing and show me the ropes of the new school like I'd seen in so many "Afterschool Specials," but that didn't happen. No one came, not even the ugly-duckling, unpopular bookworm kid that I saw on the same shows. So I spent the first year of my Junior High days in quiet anonymity, and I spent my nights alone.

I was content with the arrangement. Because I didn't know better, I thought all the other kids at Nokomis went straight home after class and stayed there until the next school day. And I grew comfortable with the way the Burton household ran. The unwritten law of the house was that my dad spent each evening in the corner living room chair, under the lamp, reading the newspaper. Although I could do as I pleased — watch TV, listen to the stereo, write or find a game to play — I was not to disturb my dad until evening's end. After that I would say goodnight and go to bed. Once I was in bed, my dad would put down his paper, make his lunch for the next day, then secured the house by closing windows, locking doors and pulling down shades.

I didn't understand the laws of school kid interaction, or even how to get along with my own family, but I knew how the evening was supposed to work in the Burton house. So my passage to adulthood didn't involve exerting my independence, becoming popular, or taking up smoking. After about a year of Junior High, I was going to be a man by taking over, or at least helping with, dad's locking up chores. Even though the job couldn't be easier, I thought my dad might even be a little proud of me for doing it. Like a private eye on a stake-out, I made note of every little thing he did: open front door and turn knob from the outside to make sure it's locked; check the window locks; take out the garbage if it's full. After months of observing, I was ready for the job. So one night I forced myself to stay up late. My dad, however, wanted to get to bed. Having finished the paper he was doing fidgety things around the house such as reorganizing the dishes in the dishwasher, getting the garbage ready to be taken out. He didn't say anything, but that was my cue to go upstairs to bed. I stuck it out though, reading the paper and playing solitaire at the kitchen table. Finally my dad gave in and said he was going to bed. When his door finally closed, I assumed charge of the house. Confidently, I set right to work checking that all the doors were locked, windows shut securely and the messes in the kitchen were picked up. When I was satisfied with my job, I went to bed.

Within ten minutes, I heard my dad get back up again and I could tell by the sound of his steps that he was going through his nightly ritual of locking up. "But I just *did* that!" I thought to myself. "What is he doing? He doesn't even..." Then the truth hit me, "He doesn't *trust* me: He won't even let me lock the house. He doesn't trust me, not even a little." The easiest job on the planet next to Vanna White's and my dad didn't trust me with it. I was shattered and began to cry. The pain of my tears said it wasn't just my dad getting up again that I cried about, but that this was the last straw. A lifetime of memories joined together like pieces of a jigsaw puzzle. "He didn't let me touch that saw when I was nine either!" I recalled. "Mark Olson was my best friend and he's gone! I'm afraid of girls. I don't belong in this family. I'm scared to go on." Then I returned to where I started: "He doesn't trust me!" They were all terrible revelations. I wanted so badly to show I could be responsible, and I was undermined by my dad's silent statement. I'd held in my feelings for so long I had to burst sometime. The tears came in such uncontrollable waves they almost felt like laughter. I had never cried that hard at any other point in my life. I cried until my teeth hurt. All the pain, all the tears and fears had buried me and suddenly, within it all, I meant absolutely nothing. As I cried I saw my whole existence before me. I saw that I could do nothing in my life and that I never *would* do anything. I *was* nothing. Almost mystically, my world fell apart that night. As trivial of an event as it would seem to anyone else, I felt that moment had ended my existence, that, in a sense, I had died.

Not only did I die, but it seemed as if I kept dying. It was fascinating because, ironically, I was living my death: I was alive and dying at the same time. There was a small pleasure underneath the pain which kept me from nearing suicidal thoughts. At that moment I felt I was the most insignificant thing in the universe, yet the pleasure came from the inescapable fact that, although I was insignificant, I was still alive. Those thoughts made me cry then stop, then cry all over again, finally crying myself to sleep that night.

Waking the next morning, I was witness to nothing less than a miracle. After getting up and walking downstairs, I'd pushed open the stairway door and was amazed to find out that everything was okay, that nothing had changed. Dad was in the kitchen cracking open a soft boiled egg like he always did before work, the morning paper was there on the table. "Wait a minute," I thought. "I died last night. I lost everything I'd ever known. What happened?" I thought the laws of physics must have somehow been broken. I was still the same as I was before last night, Dad was still the same, and the world hadn't spun off its axis. Life went on and I was still part of it. It was a divine revelation that balanced the previous night's awful revelation of having no place. In a real sense, it was a rebirth.

For the next couple of years, that taste of life and death left me crying almost every evening, dying and living each time. Like my dad shutting down the house, it became my ritual. Mostly I cried for myself, but eventually I cried also for the other kids at school who, I reasoned, must sometimes feel the same as I did. I cried for those who had even less than I did, less of a family, less freedom to cry. I cried, too, for the kids who seemed to have it all. I was afraid that their lives were passing them by and they didn't even know it. But I also realized that I wished I were like them and, until I could be, they would pass *me* by. I'd lay on my bed each evening, my head almost out the window, staring into the darkness wondering what would become of me. "Why am I here?" I would wonder in bewilderment. Then, in almost the same thought, "Why not?" Then the tears flowed because I didn't understand. And not understanding made me cry.

The ritual continued into my college years when I could often found lying on my bedroom floor with my legs folded comfortably on the bed, blasting my stereo and listening to Bruce Springsteen sing about a special kind of loneliness, of missed connections and of looking for a place. To his music, I would lie down and cry so hard I couldn't think.

Oh those barefoot street boys they left their homes for the woods
Those little barefoot street boys they say homes ain't no good
They're at the corner
Threw away all of their switchblades knives
And kissed each other goodbye

To me, that scream of tears and pain was healing.

A few years after that, except for occasional moments, I never cried with the same impact or the same passionate release again. After turning 21, I didn't cry at all. I'd wanted to and thought I should, but I coudn't simply call up the tears. It would be like trying to make myself love someone or trying to dream a special dream. The tears would have to come to me; I couldn't go to them. So by the time I had cancer, I couldn't cry because, having wept for over half of my life, I was all cried out.

At least I thought I was done. Having accepted the absence of tears in my life, I turned instead to humor. Laughing and crying were so similar they felt like the same release — and I could control my laughter. Just when I thought laughter was all I would get for the rest of my days, I had one last freeing cry. Although it wasn't the same revelatoy cries of my youth, it did cut my emotions loose and remind me that the pain was still in me.

I was on the phone with my sister, Debby. After learning I had a tumor, but before my bone transplant and the diagnosis of cancer, we talked about the strange turns in Cheryl's and my lives. Neither of us remember what brought it out, but somewhere in that conversation, and with no warning, I started to cry. It came from a sense of frustration and went back to not knowing my place in the world. It could have been a fear of dying — or of cancer. It could have been a rekindling of those junior high thoughts or the fear of justifying my life. I remember saying to her over and over, "I'm sorry, I'm sorry." And I remember wondering what I was so sorry about. For crying on the phone? For being afraid? For not having friends? For not being a better father? It must have been tears for all of that — the tears for my whole life. Maybe I couldn't be sorry enough for all that I'd done and been and for her having sit and listen to me being sorry.

Those tears had come seemingly at random. I didn't even know I had cancer then; I just knew I was afraid. But even though I didn't shed another tear again, I was glad I had both laughter and tears in me. And that was when I was thrown another curveball. Near the middle of my treatments, I caught a blood infection and went into the hospital for the harshest struggle of my life. It was the one time throughout my entire cancer when I believed I was close to dying. I was not only afraid, I was beyond desperation, I couldn't laugh or cry.

At that time I might have truly lost my humanity. Maybe all my emotions died like my soul did years ago, but if they did, they didn't return the next day, stronger than before. It was closer to the night I had gone insane on our livingroom floor and Cheryl rubbed my arms and read to me, only it lasted more than a night. It was seven more days in the hospital. I was between chemos and had caught the infection one day after getting out of the hospital. Although we never found out what caused my cancer, that infection was easily traced to my own stupidity. Never quite appreciating the phrase "take it easy" or understanding the importance of my infection-fighting white cells — which were depleted by chemo — I reasoned that my first day home from my fifth treatment, might be a good day to work on my chimney. It was an incompetent move. I had acted as if, when I left the hospital, I'd heard the doctor say, "Hey Scott, you have almost no germ-fighting white cells. Don't forget to hang around soot and exert yourself."

The infection seemed to come out of nowhere, like a punch when I wasn't looking. One moment I was putting the grill back into the hearth, and the next my body was uncontrollably chilled. I put a winter coat on to warm up, then another, and another. I piled blankets on top of the coats as I lay on our couch in the living room, my teeth chattering like castinets and my skin bristling as if someone had taken a cheese grater to it. I took three extra hot baths in an attempt to get warm and, somehow, bring my fever down. But they did nothing but make me really clean.

More than anything I didn't want to go back to the hospital. I imagined the fever would pass just like when I went in with a tiny temperature back during the early stages of chemo. I had spent four extra days on Masonic 3 for almost no reason at all. But my temperature was 103.5, so Cheryl coaxed me into emergency. After they had checked me in and done their preliminary testing, the infection kicked into a higher gear. On the gurney ride from emergency up to Masonic 3, I began shaking in a way I couldn't control as I grew painfully cold. By the time I reached the nurses station, my body was racked with phenomenal tension, part of me wanting to go into convulsions as the other part tried to remain perfectly stiff. It was called rigors.

At that point my white cell count was as low as it possibly could be. Technically, I may have even *owed* white cells. One of the doctors said they planned to keep me for another two weeks and every hope in my body fled. Initially I fought with her, contending that she was wrong about keeping me in the hospital the last time I had slight temperature, but she didn't bend. She, too, didn't trust me. Through it all, there were no tears, just a silent, burning rage. Since I hadn't eaten the entire previous week in chemo, I wondered how was I going to make it through two more. Emotionally, I sank lower and lower. I didn't have the will to laugh, cry, talk or see anyone. It was the worst thing that could have happened yet I did nothing to make it better. I stopped arguing with my doctor and just lay in my bed waiting for the week — or my life — to be over..

Family members on the phone tried to cheer me up. "It'll just be a couple weeks, Scott." "At least you're not getting chemo." "Think of the others who are suffering worse than you are." But I didn't care. I knew there were others worse off, but I couldn't think of them at all — only myself. I was miserable and that was as far as I could see. Perhaps only those who've gone through the same kind of misery could understand it, but there was no possible way to put a good face on being in the hospital. My mind said the despair would never go away and I *wanted* to hate it.

The only satisfaction I got was a call from a high school friend, Bruce Carlson. I told him how I felt and explained how I wanted to feel awful and deny my life but that no one would let me. Bruce simply agreed. He went on to say how he thought that made perfect sense. "I don't see why you should feel any better, " he said, which made me finally feel validated. "Yeah," I agreed. "There is nothing good about this. I hate my life and I hate myself. I hate the doctors. I hate the medicine. I hate the god-awful smell in this room. Gee, thanks Bruce. I feel a lot better."

Feeling better about my misery didn't make the pain go away because joy was still absent. And it wasn't that I felt better anyhow. I just felt better about hating everything. The ever present fear I carried throughout cancer of losing my humanity was stronger than ever, and on that day I talked to Bruce it became a reality. Accepting my feelings of despair, I finally got myself up to use the bathroom instead of using the metal jug I was given. It was nearly a week after I was admitted with the infection and almost two since I had eaten. When I caught sight of myself in the bathroom mirror, I was under 150 pounds (I'd started at 170), my hair was gone, my skin pasty, my body showing bones and I was still hobbling on crutches. For a split second, I didn't see myself as human. Instead, I had become a bug, a crusty, silent non-entity that was better off in a dusty corner.

Maybe that was why I didn't cry; only humans cry. Bugs do nothing but skitter around until stepped on or eaten by something. I only saw myself as an insect for a moment, but I couldn't shake the picture out of my mind. It was etched in my memory like the emotional scarring of a kid at a freak show. But even when it had passed and I was no longer a bug, I was still emotionless. The closest I got to crying was a watery-eyed whining.

After losing my humanity at the lowest point in my battle, my misery came to an end and I still was not blessed with a cathartic release of laughter or tears to wash away the pain. The whole episode, from the infection to fighting the doctors to self-loathing-turned-on-others, ended with a meal. Looking back that might have been what I needed all along. It sounds so trivial, but if I had just been able to eat something at the start I would have felt well enough to battle the infection constructively instead of destruc-tively. Maybe I would have laughed and cried. Maybe then I wouldn't have lost my humanity. But through a combination of stifling anger, bone-headed pride and a learned fear of eating in the hospital, I couldn't bring myself to ask anyone, not even my family, to bring me some outside food. It was a terrible catch-22. Not eating made me feel less human and feeling less human made me feel like I couldn't ask to eat.

It took a phone conversation with Dave for him to force me to have a meal. Regardless of my pathetic claims of, "No, that's okay, I don't think I could eat anyhow," Dave brought me some tomato soup with chips and crackers. It was like the two sides of my mind fighting again, only it was the deep inside voice in me that said, "Oh please, someone help me. Bring me some food. Take care of me" and the outside voice saying, "Nothing can help. Leave me alone." The inside voice that never made it past my lips was right all along, and when Dave brought in the basket of food, it was like being rescued after months at sea. I sat there eating and was so close to crying for joy and thankfulness at what Dave did, I was almost in awe. It was a distinctive, poignant moment for me but I still didn't cry. I don't think I even made a joke. Instead, I sat numb to the fact that, in the middle of a life-threatening illness, I almost needlessly allowed myself to die.

The next day, one week after being admitted, the doctors gave me a drug that stimulated my white cells. My white count jumped immediately leaving me wondering why they took an entire week to give me the drug. Did they think I was going to come to my senses and start enjoying my stays at the hospital? Why didn't they give it to me on the first day? For that matter, they could have given me the drug after chemo and I may have never caught the infection in the first place. But it was too late to ask those questions and I didn't want to fight with them anymore. Rose had come to my room and brought a pizza. Dave came too. I was back to joking and trying to express the deep horror of my experience with laughter and, because my white cells climbed so high, I was going home the next day. What would have been the worst two weeks of my life was, at least, cut back to one. I just wanted to go home with Cheryl. I wanted to see the kids and hear them running and being their silly selves. I wanted to sit up in our bed and hold Cheryl — or have her hold me — and cry. I wanted the tears to pour about how much I hated that week, how much I hated cancer and how much I wanted it all to be over. But there were no tears. Maybe I'll cry again someday. Or maybe I'll just end up laughing.

TV Or Not TV?

From the very beginning of my cancer battle, time was an issue. How long would it take to recover from surgery? How many months would I be in chemo? How soon before I performed again? As everything was getting more difficult, my perception of time had become altered. The second half of chemo already felt longer than the first and the blood infection made it seem like the therapy would never end. That combined with Attivan, which gave time the abstract quality of an LSD trip, only added up to a confusing framework for my recovery.

Not that time ever passed in an ordinary way at the hospital. A nine a.m. surgery meant I would be in the operating room by noon. Getting "checked right in" meant "Sit down and we'll get to you as soon as we can." And going down for a series of x-rays meant I should pack a lunch. Maybe it only held true for longer stays, but in the hospital an average 24 hour day somehow took 36 hours. Watching the sweep hand go around the clock just once took well over ten minutes. Having no charts, graphs or scientific data, I postulated that all hospitals were built in time warps just outside the laws of physics. Land was cheaper there. Plus, they got a good cable package and a cut of the parking meter money which, because of the ebb and flow of the time/space continuum, averaged out to just under $70 per minute. A time warp was the only logical explanation for the fact that, in the hospital, a visit from my family appeared to last around 10 minutes, while daily blood samples seemed to take hours. When Attivan did its job I hardly noticed. But on the occasions when I wasn't lost in Attivanland, or was between chemos, time moved with amoeba-like speed.

To combat the slowing down of time, I turned to a place where time was strictly regulated for maximum advertising dollars — the television. Sadly, because I fell off my working, writing and fitness schedule, there was nothing to do *but* watch TV. I was in a 15' x 15' hospital room where almost everything was sterile white except the pictures on the wall — and they looked like they were bought just after the store ran out of velvet Elvises and so they took what was left. All I had was a styrofoam pitcher of water, a plastic cup, plastic toothbrush, some tissues and a big metal pan for regurgitation. I would stare at the paltry pile of toiletries wishing I felt like brushing my teeth again; then I'd look to the other side of the room. In the upper corner was a big old shiny black 19" television set suspended from the ceiling that played in-house movies —and the remote control was connected right to my bed! It felt almost like a sociological experiment with the medical staff standing behind a two-way mirror saying, "What other soulless thing can we put in the room to make him turn the TV on quicker?"

Unfortunately, the price of turning on the TV to pass time was watching it. Perhaps because of the state of TV in the '90s — or maybe because of the limited reception one can get in a time warp — every channel seemed to be a direct link to the Daytime Talk Show Network. And their motto was "All Trash All The Time." I watched a nearly lethal amount of the garbage talk shows: Geraldo, Sally Jesse Raphael, Montel Williams and the like. They were shows that viewed life from its seamiest side and could have all been subtitled "National Enquirer: The TV Show." The only positive element of those shows was a built-in watchability factor for me as a chemo patient because, as opposed to the movies I watched that I ultimately felt sickened by, those shows actually *started out* by making me sick. There was no concern that, "Oh gee, perhaps I'll never feel like watching these shows again" because that was incentive.

Like car wrecks, the trash shows were impossible *not* to watch. And like a guy who charts trailer park living as a science, I became a connoisseur, the Siskel and Ebert of cheesy talk television.

"Watch, Gene, as the host paces up and down the steps of the studio with the microphone in hand, urgent as if they'd found the root of all our problems."

"I agree, Roger. And note how their eyes are stuck in a kind of pitiful concern that is a cross between provoking the audience to rage and a deep concern over how they look on video."

I had studied all of their techniques. Sally Jesse Raphael had a dim silence about her, then talked like a distant aunt who loved to pry into my life, yet she knew me no better than she knew the presidential cabinet. Geraldo was cocksure, so impressed with himself he almost couldn't stand it. He could both pander shamelessly and berate his guests at the same time. Montel Williams, on the other hand, was unsure enough of his place that he made jokes at inappropriate times and didn't seem to know if he wanted his show to be a lesson or a party. And the others, Rolanda, Jenny Jones and Jerry Springer, were at least as bad, if not worse.

Painful as it was, trash TV was a learning experience. Watching Geraldo, or Sally, or any other, it was eye-opening to see how many people in this country craved attention so desperately — and that included the *hosts* of the shows. I watched men with bodies less toned than Jabba the Hut strip nearly naked and dance for their wives. I saw mothers trying to break up their daughters' marriages and young street punks strut out on stage, proud to be ignorant of everything outside of their backwards-turned caps. I saw pimps, self-proclaimed white trash, satanists, UFO joy riders, defrocked priests, debunked doctors and a host of people claiming to be experts on everything from group sex to finding your inner child.

It was curious to me how the people on the shows dressed to fit their stereotypes. The loud-mouthed jerk redneck who maintained his right to shoot trespassers was in fact wearing cowboy boots, had a ratty beard and chewed tobacco. The over-the-hill, voluptuous sex siren who was in favor of legalized prostitution wore a low-cut black top, leather pants, Farrah Fawcett '70s hair and just enough make-up that her head tilted forward slightly. It was as if everyone came to the show direct from a Hollywood casting call.

The critic in me spoke up: "What disturbs me, Roger, is this young girl is saying she wants to be an individual, different from everyone else in the crowd (just like all her friends, I might add), but she's said the exact same thing by the demographically-typical clothes she's wearing, the mohawk, the pierced nose and heavy black eye make-up."

"Right. And she said it again with the cocky, confrontative tilt of her head, the way she sits in her chair and the smirk she gives trying to get a reaction from the crowd. This is all old hat. It's been done to death. I tell you, Gene, when I see this, I just want to scream, 'You're a one-statement human!'"

"And that statement is, 'I'm so desperate, maybe TV will help.' Now on to our next show ..."

I alternated between being disgusted by and pitying the people on the shows who maybe just needed to exorcise some demons. But it hit me that I was doing so from a hospital bed. There I was, ingesting gallons of chemo and told my odds of living were fifty-fifty, yet I felt like the fortunate one. I was sick, but I felt my life was more in balance than the lives I watched on TV. On TV, the host would be talking about a guy who still lived with his mother as if he were negotiating the hostage crisis in Iran. Maybe I had cancer, but one pathetic show after another told me there was a sickness in this country for which there isn't a cure. A weird sickness of neediness, of never having enough, of not knowing what it is to be fully content. Give me cancer any day, I thought. At least my disease was being treated. At least, as evidenced by the tube in my chest and the beeping of my IV, I *knew* I was alive.

I watched in horror one minute and the next it was so off-the-chart bad that it was funny. The things they allowed on national television were beyond ridiculous. It was as if I were getting on with my life, counting the hours, maybe brushing my teeth again and I'd think to myself, "Gee, I'll bet there isn't much of a call for left-handed cross dressers with speech impediments who have all been seen with J. Edgar Hoover." The next thing I'd know, I'd pop on the tube and see fifteen of them on a the panel of a Geraldo-type show only to find they're part of a national organization of hair-lipped, cross dressing Hooverites with a secret handshake and everything. I laughed at the things these shows passed off as entertainment, but it was the same kind of laugh as watching a politician lie through his teeth. It was laughing in pain.

It hurt not just watching the trash talk shows but watching every Hollywood insider show with the hosts slobbering over the stars, every lurid, so-called news magazines, and every commercial that implied our pathetic lives would be so much better if only we wore Michael Jordan's shoes. Everything that indirectly said, "You don't have what you're supposed to have in life, but if you listen to us, watch us and buy our products, we'll help you get through it."

Blowing all of TV's information out of the water, cancer taught the value of life. Without selling any products, cancer told me and countless other survivors that we already had everything we needed. Cancer taught, TV could only try. TV shows tried to teach what they thought was important: "10 tips for a sexy summer," "What food lowers your cholesterol," "What the 'Fonz' is doing now."

Ironically, there was a time when TV taught me something positive about life. On a small level, the sitcoms I immersed myself in during my youth showed me that anything could happen in life. They were also where I developed my comedy background. I watched the classics, "The Dick Van Dyke Show," "The Odd Couple" and "Mary Tyler Moore." I also watched many shows that were merely tile grout in the mosaic of comedy history such as "The Partridge Family," "Petticoat Junction" and "Love American Style." Watching those comedies — even the bad ones — helped me through my teenage years. They gave me a different perspective on life and, through the laughter, made me feel less alone. And I never felt as if they were trying to sell me anything — a product, an ideal or an attitude — they were just trying to be funny.

Every day after school I ran home, opened a bag of potato chips, poured a glass of milk and went downstairs to watch "Dick Van Dyke." It was like entering a whole new world. Anything and everything happened in sitcoms and that was what I liked about them. That, I thought, was closer to true life than any of the dramatic shows. Just like the trash TV I watched in chemo, real life dramas were only a facsimile, a cheap copy of what it truly is like to be alive. Back then the popular show "Family" tried to recreate what human existence was. But as cancer showed — as the best sitcoms did show — real life is the last thing you could possibly expect. Real existence is so vast, unique and limitless that we'd be fools to even try and recreate it. The TV drama could only show what a team of writers felt life was like.

Situation comedy, on the other hand, could account for any-thing and everything. The sit-com followed the full spectrum of human reactions. While I was struggling with how I should handle life, I saw a full complement of reactions from complacency to outrageousness. In the "Dick Van Dyke Show," Rob Petrie dealt with the fear of going bald by dreaming his hair fell out and grew back as a full head of cabbage. Ted Baxter, the pompous anchorman on the "Mary Tyler Moore Show," one night thought nothing of wearing a fake mustache that didn't even match the color of his hair to pretend someone else was delivering the news.   In the best sitcoms they didn't try to solve the problems of life; they just lived it. And that was how I wanted to view life. I didn't want my life to follow a set path or script. I wanted to know there were a million different things to feel and anything could happen. And, whether it was good or bad, that included cancer.

What I wouldn't give to see a survivor look at his diagnosis as if he were in a sit-com, with an anything-goes reaction. I would pay good money to see someone, upon their diagnosis, respond with excitement. I can almost see that person shout out with an ecstatic, "Yes!" while jubilantly pumping a fist, running victory laps around the office while the doctor enunciates loudly as if the patient hadn't heard correctly, "Cannn-*surrr*."

No one will ever respond that way and, realistically, no one should. I would at least like people to look at cancer in a different light though.   Nowhere was it written that cancer meant my life would fall apart or that I would soon die. I had already accepted that I was going to die anyway. And I saw that in my TV sitcom world too. On "Mary Tyler Moore," Chuckles the Clown died. Dressed as Mr. Peanut in a parade, he was shelled by a rogue elephant. On M*A*S*H, the fictional Captain Tuttle jumped out of a helicopter with everything a doctor needed — his doctor's bag, his bandages — everything except his parachute.

Sitting together with fellow survivors, I've heard more than a couple say that cancer, after their initial free fall, became the best thing that could have happened to them. It finally woke them up to what life was. So for some it was cancer that opened them up. For others it could have been the loss of a loved one, the loss of livelihood or a near-death experience.

For me it was a steady diet of "Dick Van Dyke," "The Odd Couple," "Barney Miller," "Taxi" and "Mary Tyler Moore" that helped open my eyes.

"Well Boys, It Doesn't Get Any Worse Than This"

From a small, green-carpeted, spotlit stage, the emcee plies the audience with small talk. He tells a story about feeling intimidated walking by a construction site, finishing his joke with, "It's like it had just rained testosterone before I got there." The audience can't ignore a comfortable, confident feel about him. He feels it himself, as if he knows he has nothing to lose. Folded over the top of his head, his black hair is pasted down with more than a little dab of Brylcreme. A pencil-line mustache rests above his thin lips matching the shiny black lapels running down the length of the hound's tooth jacket, and he's either chewing gum or was born with a perpetual smirk. The spotlight that makes everything off-stage look pitch black makes him look even pastier than he is. The emcee gets titters here and there from his benign patter of jokes and adjusts his tie after each one. After setting an amiable tone, the comic steps up his act and launches a joke about someone's unfashionable tie, and the crowd erupts in laughter. Some heads strain to see the tie and an energetic buzz fills the room. Pausing to let the crowd digest their communal laughter as if they've just finished a fine meal, he gives a cocky twitch of his head and realigns his tie knowing his job is done.

"Ladies and gentlemen," the emcee says, switching to a sincere tone, "coming to the stage is a very entertaining young man. He's worked with the top comics, written a script for 'Roseanne' and he headlines clubs and corporate events from coast to coast. Let's hear it for," he says, as his voice builds to a crescendo, "Scott Burton!"

Beneath the loud blast of the introduction, the audience gives up a polite entrance applause, then shuts down quietly to accentuate that it's now my turn. I jump right in, almost before the applause ends, and deliver my first joke, hoping it will set the hook so that I can spend the rest of the show reeling them in. My first line is met with absolute silence.

I'm curious as to what on earth I could have done wrong so early and what exactly they were expecting that I didn't fulfill. Thinking I may have started too fast or expected too much, I slow down and present my second joke more deliberately. The room remains stunningly quiet and I begin editing myself as I go. The third joke also falls flat, receiving blank stares and some grumbling. In desperation I make my own joke about the guy's tie. I receive even less laughter than the none I've already gotten.

I have no idea what to do next. Instead of the laughter I should be hearing, I can only hear glasses tinkling, bar blenders whirring, chairs shifting and waitresses plying their trade. The sweat begins to rush out of my pores like it's late for something, then gathers at my eyebrows when the first droplets realize, "Hey, we have nowhere to go." The eager beads of sweat rushing up from behind force the sweat already there over the top and down the side of my face. I can hear every single sound in the room and am wishing the guy in the third row would quit blinking so loud. The surrounding void distracts me, and I take an inordinate amount of time deciding what I'm going to do next. I decide to abort the mission and return to what I know best. I reach into my bag and pull out some juggling clubs. They are considered no-fail props on a comedy stage and I paste on a smile as if everything was going according to plan. I step up close to the front row to heighten the tension and perhaps draw a laugh out of the audiences fear. But I get nothing, not even nervous laughter. The people in the front row look past me as if I were only distracting their view with my act.

Attempting some initial juggling tricks, I drop consistently. The audience hardly notices because they've stopped paying attention. I see sweat droplets all over: on the front table, on my shoes, even on the lady's blouse in the front row. With each drop of a club, I instinctively make a joke about it. The tedium grows as, upon each drop, I seem to tell the same joke. The audience is restless and uncomfortable and seems ready to leave. Trying the same trick over and over, I drop over and over. The people remain stone-faced waiting for some verifiable entertainment. I'm working harder and harder, nearly *projectile* sweating, when it finally hits me. "Oh that's right," I say to myself. "I forgot, I'm not funny."

It's almost a relief to know that it was all just a mistake. Looking up I see the crowd staring at me as if they just heard every word that ran through my head. "Whoa," I say to myself, "what could I possibly have been thinking? I'm getting out of here. I wonder if Domino's is hiring."

I gather up my things apologetically, looking occasionally out to the crowd and assuming they, too, are relieved. I head toward the stage exit when the club manager calls from the side of the stage. "What are you doing?" he asks, pushing me back on stage. "You got 30 more minutes, kid. They're starting to warm up to you." I wander back to center stage to relive the anxiety and horror for an endless half hour. I'm wearing my fear like a bright orange leisure suit. If it weren't illegal, I'm quite certain, the audience would be up on stage autopsying my body to figure out why I was so bad.

That was the worst possible moment I ever had on the comedy club stage. Fortunately it was only a nightmare, something I could wake-up from and say, "Thank God it was only a dream." It was a recurring nightmare I've had for the past ten years in which everything I'd done in comedy felt fraudulent.

By the fifth week of treatment, chemo had long since taken away my ability to distinguish between dream and reality, making every experience equally as strange — real life weirder than my dreams. Even that terrible comedy club dream would have been turned on its ear had I dreamt it in chemo. After waking up, I would have gasped in relief that I was home same in bed. Stretching out and loosening my muscles, with my mind at ease, I would have told Cheryl, as she rubbed my arms, "You wouldn't believe what I just dreamt. It was the most horrendous show I've ever had. I'm so glad I'm still here with you." Then Cheryl would say, "No dear. *This* is the dream. You're still back at the club. You're not funny and the audience hates you."

That fifth week, my worst week in chemo, was no nightmare: I wasn't that lucky. It was hard core reality. If it weren't for my blood infection showing me how bad things really could be, I may not have made it. I may have assumed it was a nightmare and waited to wake up from it. Instead, as bad as things got, I felt resilient as if I had a second wind. As much as I didn't want to sometimes, I was going to live through it.

There were any number of reasons why chemo seemed extraordinarily painful that week as opposed to others. Maybe it took several doses of chemo hollowing me out that wore me away so I was more susceptible. Maybe the blood infection had me convinced that everything was worse than it really was. Maybe it was my mind's rebellion to the chemo rather than my body's that pained me. The most logical reason though was, since the pharmacist mixed my chemos fresh every week, maybe they, for some reason, upped my dosage.

Because the chemo lingered in my body, each week I went home I had a hard time eating food for a couple of days. It felt as if it coated my chest and throat so that I burned like a fire was in me until it passed. The pain I experienced that week was the worst I'd felt in the hospital So I was left for the entire week with little to do but lie in my steel-framed hospital bed watching each minute pass and knowing that every swallow would hurt. I tried to see past the pain, never quite taking my family's advice and thinking of those who had it worse than me to make me feel better. I already had concluded nothing would make me feel better. A fellow at church often encouraged me to "offer up the pain." The theory behind that was I could accept suffering as a replacement for others who suffered, to both suffer along with them and ease their suffering. As with all things supernatural there were no concrete results to be seen, but considering I had no choice but to sit and suffer, it was nice to think of someone else while doing it, and I wish I had done it more. Whereas during my blood infection I didn't do it once, during the fifth week, which was equally as traumatic, I did it a couple of times. And that was only because I learned it was okay to be miserable during my infection.

Chronic pain was weird in that, while suffering it, I'd eventually realize how long it was going to last. Then I was mentally anguished over it which brought on more pain, which caused more mental anguish and so on. During the week I had two distinct experiences. Although each pain was a unique, both opened my eyes wider than I thought they could go. Both experiences brought on hallucinations. I'm not sure if hallucinations is the right word since there were no Strawberry Fields and Lucy wasn't in the Sky with Diamonds. (Maybe Tom Bosley with a pitchfork, but no Lucy, no Yellow Submarine.) What happened was the combination of the burning pain inside and the drug-induced wanderings of my mind enabled me to actually *see* my pain. Every time I closed my eyes I saw something new, a different angle, a different level, a different version of my pain. They were represented by strange landscapes in my mind. It was beyond bizarre.

I saw these visions constantly but I remember only three. In the first one I was in the void of space. I knew it was space because I felt the silent breath of eternity on my face the same way I can feel when someone is watching me. Within the darkness, the emptiness that went on forever, were thin neon lines hanging like a wind chime, scattered loosely in no particular pattern. They looked like funky earrings or children's toys, rectangles of different sizes in the brightest colors of pink, orange, yellow and green, hanging on nothing and in nowhere.

As the pain expressed itself, the rectangle lines turned laterally one at a time, revealing a neon colored disk. Up until then I had only been seeing the edges of the disks. In no specific order they turned slowly and deliberately, then turned back before the next shape appeared. The colors seemed to scream silently as they turned, hot pink and lime green. I couldn't follow them or their irregular pattern, and their unrelenting steadiness made me anxious and afraid.

It took only a blink of an eye for a new experience to come. I opened my eyes after the first experience and found that the vision in my head wasn't surreal: My room was. The stark white sheets contrasting the painful black in my head, the metal spit pan on my lap, the burn and effort of every swallow, even the fact that I occupied physical space seemed odd. I was between two worlds without belonging to either one. Because I couldn't help it I closed my eyes again and the next thing I knew I was hovering above an otherworldly, lunar landscape. I wasn't in the picture, nor was it me flying over the rocky terrain. I was the pictures I was seeing. *I* was the turning neon discs, *I* was the empty void of space.

In the second vision I was the craggy rocks I hovered above. Not individual rocks but rather one large, unnaturally textured rock. It was rusted orange with such obtuse structure I could imagine the pinching in my feet to walk on it. It was like the lava rocks used for gas grills if Salvador Dali had gotten ahold of them and breathed a tiny, tortured life into each pore. They were frighteningly unreal. Sometimes it was as if my presence was rolling along the mutated rocks like a child rolls down a grassy hill. I had no control or orientation. Also, because it wasn't me flying, it was like the feeling of being in one of those Omni or Imax surround theaters where, if the camera is in a plane, you feel every rise and fall of it. Again, as I patrolled dizzyingly over the rocky scene, I *was* it. My view focused with increasing clarity to the point where I wouldn't think they could get any clearer and then I would somehow focus in deeper and sharper. I could feel it.

The visions were so unreal I wanted to write them down so I'd never forget them. Initially I had planned to write about the colored disks — a poem or a story that, for me, would always convey the eerie feeling of both the vision and the week. But before I wrote anything down, I had another vision similar to the first. In this one I was in space again, but everything was heavy and moved slowly as if through syrup. Everything was black, and I felt myself, or maybe it was something else, drop through down an endless chasm. I couldn't get out of my head the insane quiet with which it dropped. As opposed to the others, this vision held an air of mysticism about it. The experience was so frighteningly beautiful and profound that I wrote about it.

The Pearl

It drops.
Not a pearl.
Not a black pearl.
But a black pearl nonetheless.

Through the ocean stillness of silence
that is inside me,
inside my head,
my inner head.
Dropping to the core, the base of my neck and spine.
Perfectly liquid.

A perfectly still ocean
ceasing of cold, ceasing of motion,
ceasing of touch
(but the drop of a pearl),
ceasing of all until it is air,
but black water still.

And that pearl went to hell.
So silent a journey I would not have thought.
And she became there.
The brightest red lips, her cheeks curved to a marble chin,
her stoic ocean green eyes, her hair pulled back black tight
to reveal all her temptuous beauty ...
and sorrow ... and purity.

Her face
was larger than the pearl,
larger than me.
And I dropped,
we dropped (the pearl and I),
silently to hell.
And this time I could hear the drop.

And it was silent.

I don't know what the poem means or what any of my visions meant. Interpreting them would be like trying to explain smiling, or sleep, or death. But they all made an impression. They all said something, and that defined me for most of my fifth week.

I could have never expected it, but there was a second leg to that week that would add irony and a completely different kind of pain. Maybe it was because of my ongoing visions, or the brutal dosage I was receiving or my lack of humor, but I began feeling terribly emotional on my fifth day. I had talked to Rose earlier that day and though I usually don't call someone without any reason in mind, I felt it was vitally important to call Jack in Los Angeles. If nothing else I just needed to tell him I loved him; I wanted to call everybody and say the same thing.

I talked quietly and was close to tears. Usually I like to be vibrant on the phone, especially when talking to Jack because, contrary to how he feels about himself, I've always seen him as a ray of hope.

"Hello?" Jack answered.

"Hi, Jack. How're you doing?" I said sadly.

"I'm fine. You don't sound so great. How are you?"

"I don't know. I just felt like I really had to call. I just really wanted to let you know that I loved you."

"I love you too, Scott." Then there was a brief pause. "I'm sorry about Cheryl's mom."

The words sounded awful before I even knew what they meant. My heart dropped.

"What do you mean? What happened?"

"She died. You didn't know?"

When I'd talked to Rose, she gave me the impression that all was well. I was so confused and emotionally lost that I didn't know what to say. After hanging up with Jack, I called her back asking why she said everything was fine. "Everything *was* fine," she maintained.

"That's not what Jack said," I replied, hoping maybe Jack was wrong. Rose finally admitted what was going on. Everyone had instructions from Cheryl not to tell me about her mother while I was in chemo because she didn't think I would be able to handle it. And she was right.

Eventually Cheryl told me the whole story. At a stop sign on a rural road, her mother, Elizabeth Conway, pulled out over the crossroad when a large semi-trailer, whose driver later said his brakes weren't working properly, ran through his stop sign into her car, killing her instantly. I could only stand in utter silence. The suddenness of the loss was completely numbing.

The irony was enraging. What awful irony that so many, even Betty, were so heavily concerned about *my* well being. What could be said? What could even be *thought?*

My body grew shaky from fear. I don't remember if I was on crutches or in a wheelchair, but I got myself out to the nurses station. Having no idea what I could do, I explained the situation and said I needed to go home immediately. But since it was over, there was nothing I could do except try to comfort Cheryl, and I was in a poor position to do that.

Cheryl was gone anyway. The wake was that weekend in Baraboo, Wisconsin, where Betty grew up. Cheryl strongly and confidently walked into the situation. The funeral was where the grace that was with her from the start blossomed. She was assured, deep at the core of her soul, that her mother was taken care of. There was, and still is, no doubt in her mind that Elizabeth Grace Conway had found heaven. Elizabeth Grace. Was that the grace that Cheryl was given?

I've heard others talk about lost loved ones. They put on their best faces and say, "I know she's in a better place." But so often the uncertainty shows through. Cheryl is even one of those who can spot that self-doubt in others. But in her it simply didn't exist.

Cheryl never had the relationship with her family that she wanted. She was in the midst of patching up a severed relationship with her mother. As far back as she can remember, her dad seemed distant, angry and didn't communicate his love towards her. Her relationship with her brother was also painful and even diminished what joy she had in childhood. At that particular moment, the death of her mother, there was no reason for her to find peace, yet she had. Cheryl said she felt the presence of Mary and believed that was the source of her peace. That may be true, but I feel another source of her peace was her special gift of grace.

Despite the backdrop of sadness and death, it was a blessed weekend for Cheryl. Along with the peace she felt about her mother, while riding to the wake with her estranged father, she suddenly saw him with new eyes, maybe a new heart. As they drove he revealed something quiet and lovable about himself, a fragileness that he hadn't shown to her before. He talked about things he wished he'd done and of things he'd like to do. After that, she wanted the chance to communicate with him again and re-kindle their lost relationship. She also saw her brother in a new way. Their past would never be totally erased, but she finally saw him for what he was, an intelligent grown man, a husband and father and a sensitive human being who suffered pains in his childhood himself.

Betty's death was dumbfounding and painfully non-negotiable and showed us all the cruelest cycle of life. But somewhere, alongside their great loss, there was a gain. For a brief moment, while in the state of grace, Cheryl saw her father, brother and herself as a family. A need grew that was never present before and her dad and brother felt it too. There is, however, no rosy ending: They have since drifted apart again. But there was a moment of rebirth, a glimpse of what still can be.

The frustrating part of the experience for me, was that I couldn't be part of it. I was still in chemo at the time insisting to the nurses that I had to go home. I must admit, part of my insistence was that I just wanted to leave chemo, but I also felt the need to be home. Even though Cheryl wasn't there and I couldn't comfort her, I needed to be in a familiar place where I could reflect on what had occurred.

The nurses granted my wish but not immediately. I had a full day of chemo left so what they did was speed up the drip on my IV bag and let me receive a full day's worth of chemo in about a half day. That sounded attractive at first, but then I realized I already struggled more than usual with this particular chemo. Although I was afraid a speeded up dose might cause even more trouble, we went ahead with it anyhow.

My family decided that in my state, I shouldn't be left alone for the night. Personally, I didn't understand why that had to be, but at the time I didn't understand much of anything. I didn't understand simple conversation, why the hospital sheets were white or why people kept calling me "Scott." Decisions weren't best left to me and part of me knew that. So Arlene nominated herself to be the one to spend the night with me in my hospital room.

Everyone knew how badly I was handling chemo, and with the speeded up dosage we looked for a proper drug to help me cope. The logical choice was Marinol — marijuana in pill form. Unfortunately I took a Marinol pill once earlier and it made me throw up so horribly that I'm still emotionally scarred and gag whenever I think of it. Since pill form was out, the other option was the good old illegal route. My family left that decision to me, and I figured, I was in no position to care what I took. "If it'll help, why not," I said.

The only question was how to get it. The nurses didn't keep any of the non-pill drug handy (or, if they did, it wasn't for the patients). But Dave, being more familiar with the roll-your-own drug world than the medicinal one, was at the ready. After we'd decided to use the illegal drug, he was out the door in a shot. "Give me half an hour," he said. "I'm sure I can find good quality."

Within half an hour, he was back in the room with some nicely wrapped packages of cannabis weed. It must have been close to evening by then because the next thing I remembered was lighting up, me in my bed, Arlene in one of those ugly vinyl chairs that seemed uncomfortable by design.

In a week in which everything was off-the-wall or insane, Arlene and me sharing a joint was the perfect topper. Arlene, although she had dabbled in illegal smoke in her younger days, is one of the most straight-laced women you're likely to find. And I, while not being as morally pure as she, had never tried marijuana or any other drug before. We were like a couple of junior high school kids learning how to smoke.

Without noticing the lack of pain, I was convinced the drug had no effect on me. My mind felt the same as it always did. I certainly didn't feel loopy or anything. Just as I was telling Arlene that Dave gave us inferior stuff, my usual night nurse, Kitty, came in and said there was something different about me. I couldn't believe she didn't already recognize the distinct odor of a Grateful Dead concert or a Cheech and Chong film festival, but Arlene and I told her what we were up to. Kitty said, without a hint of sarcasm, "I can tell I'm seeing the real you for the first time."

Kitty might have been right, or it could have been the effects of Betty's death that made me sober enough for her to say that. Either way, I made it through the night and left chemo early the next day. As I was dropped off at my empty home, it struck me odd that on the same day I was given worse news than that of my own diagnosis, I tried pot for the first time.

So much happened that week. Everything that occurred followed a thread of strangeness: the delusions, the horrible accident, the Attivan, the marijuana, Cheryl's peace and grace, Arlene's comfort, Kitty's comment. It was as if none of it should have happened, yet all of it did, the most profound moment being when Cheryl's mother died. And, like wanting to record my delusional wanderings, her passing I can never forget.

o order copies of **A Life in the Balance** --

ail to Scott Burton @ Inconvenience Productions

     P.O. Box 581083, Minneapolis, MN 55458

ease send __ copies of **A Life in the Balance**
$12.00 plus $1.50 per book postage to

☐ Mr.   ☐ Mrs.   ☐ Ms._____

ddress_____

ty_____ State_____ Zip_____

t can also be ordered through your local Barnes &
oble or Borders bookstore)

Unfortunately, I have no marketing campaign
or large publisher behind this book to sell it.
The only way it can get to the public is by
word of mouth. So, if you enjoy this book or
find it worthwhile, please recommend it to
your friends, pass along this order form, or
visit my web site at: **http://www.sburton.com**
(email: scott@sburton.com)   Thanks.

Buddy Can You Spare a Nap?

Even more so than usual, after the fifth week of chemo, there was no better feeling than going home. I still couldn't eat for a day or so, but that wasn't the point. Although Cheryl was still at the wake and the kids were being baby-sat, seeing the familiar walls and getting to walk around in my own home felt like a luxury. The three week spans between chemos were like entire summer vacations, but after the surreal fifth chemo, I was like Alice returning from Wonderland. The pleasures of home were real, not imaginary. And not only was I home again, I was more than halfway done with my treatments.

Almost being done with chemo posed an unusual problem: What was I going to do with my life once it was returned to me? I hadn't worried about that for so long because I hadn't needed to. For months I could simply assume my life would never be back in my own hands and there was a weird comfort in that. Though I was taking toxic, mind-altering chemicals and my life had basically shut down, I had grown so used to my dependency on the hospital that I couldn't imagine anything different. It was like staying in an abusive relationship because I didn't know what else to do.

Adapting to life in chemo was a series of stages and I was in the last one. It began when I had my allograph and first treatments. I was anxious but almost a bit excited about what it would all be like; I wasn't concerned with how long fighting cancer would take or even the pain I'd go through. I was like a kid with my first dollar in a small town drugstore, intimidated and impressed by all the merchandise and staff but naively confident because I had a *whole* dollar.

Once I had a taste of what chemo was really like, however, I wasn't a fresh kid anymore. During the next stage I saw the drugstore for what it really was and prepared myself for the long haul. The salespeople were going to try and sell me stuff I didn't want, and I had to ignore, even mistrust them. With open eyes I became an idealistic young socialist thumbing my nose at the capitalistic drugstore, bucking their system, playing by their rules only until I was strong enough to change their outdated philosophies.

Then, with hardly a warning, chemo began to affect me in ways I never expected, confusing my mind, hollowing out my insides and making it painful for others to see me. At that stage I was no longer young, fresh or idealistic — I was a survivor. I became the old guy who sits outside the drugstore on a bench, drinking orange pop out of a bottle and telling pointless stories. I was a crusty old guy just dying to run into some young fellow going in for chemo for the first time who talked about shaving his head and growing a beard so I could say, "You ain't growing nothin'."

The stage I was now entering signaled that the long haul was coming to a close, but left me unsure of what would happen next. Would I live or die? Would I juggle again? Would my life go back to normal and what *was* normal? At this point I became the 95-year-old druggist behind the counter who had lost his memory and looked like a tired George Burns saying, "I can't remember ever not having this job."

I couldn't imagine starting my life over, especially after what I'd gone through. Did Neil Armstrong fit right back into society after walking on the moon? I told Bill Arnold and another comic friend, David Wood, when they'd taken me to lunch one day, how unsure I was of fitting in. "What will I do when this is all over?" I asked. "Will I still do comedy? *Should* I still do comedy?" They reassured me that there were many directions I could go in life: returning to comedy, writing or public speaking. Which direction I went wasn't the issue though; the key was to believe in whatever direction I went. David confidently told me that whatever it was that I was supposed to do after cancer would make itself apparent, and I would know because I would do it with passion.

There was a game I played that helped prepare for my life going any direction. Even before I had cancer, I'd look at everyday normal people and create histories for them. On the outside they'd look completely normal, but I'd picture them as skydivers, loan sharks or people living secret lives. Maybe my bus driver was a Holocaust survivor. Maybe my waitress has a gambling problem. My assumption of other people's histories reminded me that everyone has been through something, that I'm not the only one.

At the post office downtown, for example, while checking my mail I couldn't help but watch people walking down the long corridor and wonder about their lives and how they fit in. "Look at that guy," I'd mutter to myself. "He's not on crutches, I wonder what he does with his life. I wonder if he's had cancer. Hmmm, maybe he had something else. Maybe he has AIDS right now. He doesn't look like he's worrying about what's next. He's getting on with his life, visiting the post office as if nothing's wrong. Wow! Who knows?" my mind would ramble. "Maybe he's a Vietnam vet. I'll bet those aren't even his own legs. Probably some tragic shrapnel accident and yet he's found his purpose and is fully productive, maybe an executive or a self-made businessman. Boy, you sure got to admire someone like that. Well, if he can do it, why not me?"

So while virtually manufacturing the pasts of others, from the woman whom I convinced myself had cleaned houses until she became a neurosurgeon to the former trapeze artist who recently had a hip replacement and became a famous painter, I found inspiration in those around me to take comfort in wherever my life would go. "Who am I, " I thought, "to let down an AIDS infected war veteran with no legs who sells his own hand-made pottery to support the twelve adopted kids he rescued from the streets." Not only did the game inspire me, but it made me feel closer to the people I watched.

Since my junior high years I'd believed struggle was what life was all about, yet I was comforted to see it in action. Whether real or imagined, the struggles of others gave me peace in mine because it meant I wasn't alone. Who knows, maybe seeing my struggle gave others the same kind of assurance in their lives. Perhaps as I was creating scenarios for others in the post office, the lady delivering packages was thinking to herself, "Gee, it's sure nice to see that bald guy on crutches with the leg brace out and about and not home feeling sorry for himself. That shows initiative. It's too bad he talks to himself so much though. I wonder if he carries a gun. Hmmm, I'd better hurry on back to the car."

Having cancer meant I would start again from square one. That wasn't anything new. In my eyes, every new day for anyone is starting from scratch. Every day can be a brand new world of untold joy or life-altering trials or anything in between. That was what made life exciting for me — that it could be anything at any moment. It's not the popular definition of the phrase but, for me, it was living in the now. As I'd heard in a Van Morrison song, and later in church in a Bible passage, "We live and move and have our being." That is living in the now. And while I took some comfort in that idea, at that point in my treatments, I wasn't so sure who or what my being was.

The common idea of living in the now is only seeing the present and not thinking one bit about tomorrow or yesterday. Maybe I don't understand it fully because that sounds a little ignorant to me, but my version involves a lot of the past and present. I'm probably better off leaving this kind of thinking to Shirley MacLaine, but it seems to me that each moment I live, while being vital in and of itself, is also dependent on the past and the future. Without the past I never would have reached the moment that I call the present, and without the future there would be no other moment to call now. To me they all blend together. By process of elimination, my definition of living in the now is not living in the past or only for the future. It's like a 3-D picture where all time co-exists, but you can only focus on one thing at a time. So for me, even though I was aware of the past and future, I made the attempt to embrace each moment until the next one came along. I lived one day at a time keeping in mind I still had a house payment to make.

I can't say I always practiced what I preached. I still found time to complain, whine and spout off about everything from the med students' early rounds to not wanting anymore drugs. I altered my definition of the now to accommodate my nature — I lived, moved, *complained* and had my being. So I'd worry, be happy for each moment, return from chemo to be with Cheryl, wonder where we'd get money, watch the kids, drive around and worry some more. I did a little bit of everything, living for the now, living for forever. The only thing I missed out on during all that time was sleep.

I hadn't had a consistent good night's sleep for the past 15 years. The same obsessive kind of logic that defined what it was to live in the now kept me awake at night. With cancer I had a new subject to dissect in my head. I was in a catch-22. Although lying in bed was the best, quietest time for thinking, thinking was the very thing that kept me from sleeping. Tired from a day's work and no sleep the night before, I'd find myself in bed thinking, "Wow, I'm tired. I am so tired my body could legally be declared bone-dead. I can't believe how tired I am." Then I'd think, "But, if I'm so tired, how come I'm awake now? Why am I thinking about making Rachel's lunch tomorrow? Why am I thinking about what joke I should start my show with? Why am I thinking about that article I wanted to write? Maybe I'm *not* tired. Maybe I should be writing, or planning something or doing something. I should be too tired to even think 'why am I still awake?'" I then spend another two hours thinking about what I could do if I weren't so tired. Then, once I had distracted myself from wondering why I was still awake, I'd finally fall asleep.

In chemo there were a couple of weeks I don't remember being awake at all, but during the others I don't remember a peaceful sleep. Whether in the hospital or at home I hoped my being so tired from chemo would knock me out no matter what was on my mind, but it didn't happen. In the hospital they sometimes gave me two or three sleeping pills an evening and I still couldn't fall asleep. I usually didn't ask for pills because Cheryl drove it into my head that, if I ever relied on sleeping pills, I would be addicted for life. I would spend all our money on hundreds of prescriptions, ignore the family and my work, end up on the street, unshaven and in rags bumming Tums off people coming out of pharmacies. So I didn't take sleep aids often.

I remember once being surprised by how long it took for a sleeping pill to work. Not being familiar with the drug, if it didn't knock me out within the first minute I thought it took a lot of gall calling it a sleeping pill. "Those drug companies do it on purpose," I thought after an hour of remaining awake. "They sell defects just so we have to buy more." Then I stewed about being awake for three more hours, blaming everyone from the pharmacy downstairs to the Apollo 11 crew. "What's the deal here? If nothing happens within the next two hours I'm calling the nurse." (Joe Passive-Aggressive strikes again.) At about four o'clock I rang the nurse again. "Could I get another one of those sleeping pills, please?" I asked politely. "I think maybe you grabbed the placebo container by mistake." As she got another while I stewed a little more about the first one not doing its job. An hour after taking the second pill I began to think they had no effect on me. "Immunity to sleeping pills may be my secret power," I concluded. It wasn't that great of a power. I was no Spider-man or Green Lantern. It wasn't like I could get myself a cape and start fighting crime: **Attivanman, staying awake for truth, justice and the American way. Attivanman's mystical powers attained through a chemo experiment gone awry enable him to wait up until the nation's criminals fall asleep. Then, defiantly, and without regard to personal safety, Attivanman sneaks away and calls the police.**

While daydreaming of superhuman powers and trying to make pictures out of the designs on the ceiling tile in the darkness, I saw that it was almost six in the morning. I finally decided the new pill wasn't going to work either, and, just as I was about to call the nurse again, I nodded off. So technically the pill *did* work.

I had the same problem sleeping at home. (But knowing she wouldn't want to make the drive, I didn't call the nurse.) Taking matters into my own hands, I stood next to the medicine cabinet with the little pill in my hand, looking at it with contempt. The pill just sat there smugly, not saying anything as usual. But I knew it wasn't the pill's fault anyhow because in college I'd conditioned myself not to sleep. I used to stay up late every night and never fell the worse for it. On the contrary, the quiet of the night and the absence of business made it the perfect time for being awake and thinking. During those times I wrote, thought endlessly about my past and about who I was. I've kept myself up for more than a decade wanting to use that quality time the same way I used to, but my body can't handle that schedule anymore.

The massive doses of Attivan in my IV were better than the pills, usually letting me sleep before morning. Even in chemo, I thought of the sleepless nights as opportunities for quality thinking or writing. Most of these late nights ended without the payoff of a wonderful thought, only a painfully tired head the next day. But I remember one night that rekindled the excitement of my past late night activity. It was the feeling that I embraced in my college days and had clung to every sleepless night since then.

That night I was blessed with a visit that nearly raised my spirits to the heavens. Before the visit I was fidgety and antsy about not sleeping the night before, as if I had much to say but no one to say it to. Then in came Cheryl along with two of my sisters, Debby and Rose, and Debby's stepdaughter Marnie. They must have been having a good time together because they came in laughing and full of smiles, emanating love and joy. It was magical, as if every secret to life, every possible meaning was wrapped up in their smiles, in their glowing faces and their simple presence.

Before any of them had said a word, my emotions had soared. From the moment they entered the doorway, I could feel their energy. I grew hopeful and almost giddy. I was as excited as a frisky terrier when its family comes home after being on vacation for a week — except there were substantially fewer messes on my floor. Rose pulled up a chair and asked me how I was doing, remarking that my skin was a more attractive shade of pale. Debby laughed, slightly embarrassed, and apologized in case Rose's remark seemed offensive. Then she agreed that I did look better, adding, "Did you get a haircut?" We all laughed, me the most, because it was so apparent we were all equal. Because they didn't treat me like I was in chemo, I didn't feel like I was in chemo. In the same way as the nurse who told me I was going to be shiny, they treated me like a human being. They came to visit a good friend as if they were stopping at a neighborhood bar, not out of concern that he was going die. We shared each other's energy, and, even though I don't remember much of what we talked about, it was a profound kind of communication — a communication of understood love. That was how I knew that to truly live in the present there had to be knowledge of the past and future.

The girls' visit made me flash me back to Sunday dinners, years ago, at the Burton home. Those were occasions where jokes and irreverent banter flew around the table as fast as the roast beef and mashed potatoes. Mockeries, smart talk, questions, valid points on important issues — all the talk solidified one thing: We were all equal. From Debby, who usually held court, to Jack, who was the funniest, all the way down the line, we were all a part of the same experience. Those years became present and real to me again. Then, in another flash, I fast forwarded back to my hospital room, my sisters and niece sharing their lives all over again with me.

Even after they left, I couldn't forget the energy they infused me with or how beautiful their faces were. That night, when the sleeplessness came back, I was ready for it. And, as I did in my youth, I could focus on everything, not just one thing at a time. I saw my father holding Arlene when she was a baby. I saw Cheryl and me riding my motorcycle when we were courting. I saw the mountains of snow outside our Minneapolis home in winter. I saw my family grow up and my kids being born. I saw all the tears I'd cried and wished I could cry all over again. I saw people and places I had never seen before, only heard about. I saw forever.

Although Cheryl is the poet in the family, I spent that entire night and most of the morning writing and rewriting a poem. Even as I wrote it I felt it was childish in its approach and that its cadence was anything but poetic. Yet I love it and loved writing it because it was exactly how I felt.

A Love Poem

I love this life.
Maybe because I'm getting out of chemo tomorrow.
Maybe it's because I see an end to this cancer.
Maybe just the right news at the right time revived my spirit.
I want to talk about it forever.

I want to gab incessantly until it's not even words spoken
but gestures,
and eyes spreading wide, chests filling with air and arms
tense with excitement.
I want to gab, not even about the profound,
but of the love, the love of this family,
of football at the creek with kids we don't see anymore,
of the War Memorial Blood Bank, car deals, children's songs and minds.

I want to lay you all in my arms Cheryl and Marnie and Rose and Debby,
Jack, Arlene and David.
I want you all in my arms.
And I want to sing
laying on my back and you all laying upon me.
I want to sing a song that makes me cry
from the top of my head,
because my head is so far from me
in a place where tears mean something different and untouchable

(Not from my heart because my heart is with you).
But I want the song to be sung specifically to each of you
not all of you. Only something you can hear.
Cry to you all and sing to you all. Bryan and Fabi,
Judy and Brent.
I don't want to laugh because to cry and sing is to laugh.
To laugh is all I am.
I want to sign a beautiful song to my deaf parents.

And the things that I touch I want you to touch,
the back of a chair, my juggling equipment,
stones I dig my hands into
in the front yard,
and especially the air.
To bring my hand up and grasp, to
bring down the whole existence of my life
in my palm, in particles blown from eternity and God's nostrils.
I can't squeeze myself hard enough.
Squeeze me, all of you, hard enough
until I lose my breath
and I'll fall fainten in full joy
in Nirvana, Shangri-la
and eternal Holy Heaven.

That is a death I will take as it is,
a death of the grandest life.
Because from that I will get up
and live again.

After reading and re-reading that poem, I want to live it all over again. I want another sleepless night like the one I had and to feel that excitement in every second of my life. Yet, realistically, I know I can't because, if I always felt that excitement, what would I have to look forward to? I can't because my moon-eyed, summer of love looks would make people want to slap the stupid grin off my face. I can't because I would never get a job done if all I cared about was another hug.

Even though I don't get to have that feeling, I have the pleasure of having known it, of believing that someday I'll have it again and of sharing it with others. I'll carry that feeling like I carry my wallet

or my favorite book, and know it's there when I need it.
     But first — a nap.

Raising Oncologists
For Fun and Profit

Since the best feelings during cancer were my times at home between chemos, it stood to reason the worst were the times in chemo. It wasn't as bad as being under a dentist's drill for a week straight with no Novocain, but there aren't many people, survivors or not, who would argue that chemo was a good time. No one ever said to me with a smile, "You know, one day we'll look back on all this and laugh." If someone had, they would have found themselves wiping some well-aimed vomit off their shirt as I'd say, "That's okay, someday we'll laugh about *that* too."

Ironically, I *have* looked back on it and laughed. I've laughed about many of the events in chemo, and with family as well as with other survivors about their cancers. But it was never chemo itself we laughed about, it was specific moments. For instance, when my chemo spilled, the nurses dressed in radioactive-resistant garb like they were cleaning Karen Silkwood. *They* wouldn't touch the stuff but it was okay to shoot it into *my* body! Or, one week, trying to convince the nurses I was supposed to get chemo-*lite*. Or the time I changed rooms and, as I was gathering my things, the incredibly inept nurse's assistant who picked up a plastic bedpan and said in all seriousness, "Is this your hat?" They were all scary times, knowing my life hung in the balance. But, as individual moments, they were also funny. As I realized when I was a kid, there was nothing not to be afraid of — now it was chemo, cancer and the allograph — but the lighter moments reminded me that there was also nothing not to laugh about.

There were plenty of places to go for a good laugh, but I never had to go much further than my own backyard. A little bit at their expense, I often got a chuckle dealing with the oncologists, though not always on purpose. Amusing and entertaining are not qualities normally associated with the medical profession. "This week on Jay Leno, you've read his articles in the Harvard Journal of Medicine, seen him perform open-heart surgery on the Health Channel, and he's currently at Caesar's Palace in Las Vegas, opening for Charo, with his uproarious ventriloquism act along with his crazy little pal, Stitch, Dr. David Hoffman!" It's not likely to happen.

There are plenty of friendly, good natured and warm doctors, but for the most part, they aren't social butterflies. And oncologists are just like the rest of the medical profession but even more so. For many doctors, with their studies, clinics and huge case loads, their jobs dictate that they be slightly distant. And it amuses me that they roam the halls of a place full of emotion — a place to be anything *but* distant — and walk through looking at charts, poking and manipulating their clientele. That's like walking into a coffee shop in which everyone was stark raving naked from their scalps to their heels, ordering a latté as if nothing were odd, casually say to a nude patron, "That's an awful lot of body hair," then walk nonchalantly out.

How could they *not* want to sit and talk with every person on their floor? How could they not want to hold each person's hand and tell them it'd be all right? I suppose that was part of the problem: They couldn't. The sheer volume that they dealt in (not to mention a 4 o'clock tee time) meant they had to hustle through their business. Some did their best to connect, others didn't.

Some survivors have had wonderful relationships with their doctors. They've connected on a personal level to the point that they've trusted their physician not only with their health care but for recommending a good movie, advice on raising children, a good Vietnamese restaurant and tips on fashion sense. But I was happy with the professional relationship I had with my oncologists. My primary physician is a good example of a button-down doctor. He got to the point, was always sincere and gave me plenty of smile about watching him and his pals on their rounds.

I played the same game with the oncologists on their rounds that I did when I invented the histories of people I didn't know at the post office. With the doctors I imagined how much they could get away with if they abused their authority and power. While watching them crowd around a patient's bed, I pictured a medical mugging. It would have been easy. One of the docs would only have to shout out, "Oh my God! An aneurysm!" then motion for an intern to sneak behind him. The other doctors crowd close while the patient frantically checks his head. By then the intern would have the guy's wallet, pluck out the cash, flip the billfold over his shoulder and give a high-sign to the first doctor who would cover his tracks by saying, "Oh, sorry. I meant to say, 'An' yer name is?'"

I fluctuated between envying and mocking the doctors on my floor. I was impressed with how much they knew and the fact that, regardless of how friendly they were, they were saving people's lives. I mocked them because they got paid just under a billion dollars to do it, they didn't always do what was right for the patient and, often, it took a whole roomful of the guys to rustle up one personality between them.

Just for one week, I wish the physician's job depended not on his or her medical abilities, but on how friendly he or she was with the patients. What a new experience that would be. On my next visit to the clinic the doctor is in the examining room waiting for *me*, which would be a major abnormality. A doctor actually waiting for and greeting patients in a clinic is, I'm pretty sure, one of the first signs of Armageddon. (The *second* horseman I believe.) But there he is wearing a colorful bow tie that compliments his radiant smile. On his chartreuse lab coat there's a sticker that says "I hugged a clown today" and he extends his hand out, shaking mine vigorously, "Well, hi, Scott. Gee, it's good to see you again. Isn't this crazy weather we're having? I don't know whether to carry sunscreen or an umbrella. Ha ha ha! But you know what they say, 'if you don't like the weather in Minnesota, wait five minutes and it'll change.' Ha ha ha. That's so true."

I stare uncomfortably at him, waiting for him to stop and say, "You realize you get charged triple rates for me talking friendly with you." It's an awkward pause, but the world's friendliest oncologist presses on. "So, Scott. Or can I call you Scotty? Some of the staff indicated you're a little displeased in the hospital. Just so you know, we're planning on removing some of those bulky IV stands and life support systems to install some blackjack tables and slot machines. That ought to brighten your time with us, wouldn't you say? Hey, you might get lucky."

"Well, um, I guess. But that's not why I'm here. I've got some terrible pains in my chest and I don't know what they are. And about the hospital, I was just wondering if my insurance would cover my blood infection stay."

"Wow. I see you're really dealing with some issues here. I want you to know, I *feel* your pain. I tell you what, before we move on to the medical stuff, what do you say we have a cup of cappuccino and discuss our feelings. Say, would you like me to rub your back?"

Maybe someday a gregarious and involved doctor will be the norm, but I was glad to have any relationship as long as I could trust them. Yet it always struck me odd that, considering the time I've spent with both of my main oncologists, it's curious that we didn't have a more personal relationship. Heck, I wrote to a couple kids after summer camp, and that was only for a weekend and neither of them saved my life.

The reality was the oncologists toured the floor because they had to. Since it was my life and all, they figured, perhaps it would be a good idea to tell me where it was heading. That wasn't a bad thing as far as I was concerned, but if the doctor's intentions were bad, hurtful or misleading, that would have been a different matter. Mine were not. But just as there are people in every slice of life who use their communication skills and others who don't, or some who are hurtful and some who are not, oncologists followed the same rules. But due to the nature and demands of their jobs, oncologists were less likely to have a high percentage of extroverted communicators as opposed to, say, the Toastmasters.

I got along with all the oncologists who patrolled Masonic 3. My only heated clash was during my blood infection with one of my primary doctors. And, even then, I'm sure she only did what she truly felt was right for me. As opposed to the nurses, with whom I felt more emotional support and camaraderie, and counted on seeing the same friendly face, I didn't mind so much seeing a new oncologist every day. It was like trying a new ride at the fair — I know the ride is popular and mechanically sound, many other people have enjoyed the trip and the likelihood of my getting hurt is minimal. The only hard part is trusting the toothless guy running the machine.

Instinctively, I trusted the nurses more. I followed the doctors orders and regimens, but my ties to them weren't as strong. The whole hospital system had a corporate feel to it. The doctor was like the CEO that the employees see only once a year at the company party. He or she makes all the vital decisions — as well as a bundle of money. The CEO/doctor's decisions were passed to the nurses station, who served as middle management, then were given to my personal nurse who was my manager. The patients on the floor, filled the roles of the peon, minimum-wage hour workers.

I almost had pity for the doctors. On the material level they got all the accolades. They got big fat checks, wrote important papers and received all the credit. But in the end it was the nurses, the patients, the visitors and the family who seemed to learn the most. All the players in my real-life survival fight got a chance to grow as a result of it. The doctors who chose to see only the bottom line missed out on that growth. The ones who took the opportunity for growth couldn't always make it their highest priority. What the doctor got out of the relationship was a statistic, another mark in the win/loss column, maybe a bead on how to approach the next line-up. Since I had no choice but to look at my experience from all sides — medical, emotional and spiritual — I had a lot of potential for learning more about life. What a lot of doctors missed out on was what I and all who invested themselves into the experience got from it — a chance to be more human.

I didn't think it at the time, but maybe what's wrong with health care in general is the loss of humanity. Without the emphasis on care, what's left is only health. As a science, medicine will always be around to keep us around a little longer. But maybe, just maybe, it doesn't matter how long we keep each individual alive — a few more years or a few more days. Since we will all pass someday, what matters most is the ability to come to grips with that — finding peace with the life you have. Maybe health care, more than anything is just being there. A firm handshake can be health care and a warm hug. A smile is health care — laughing, understanding are too. Communicating with love and without fear is health care.

I got health care from Cheryl. Every time we talked in the kitchen or sat on the couch together was medicine. Every time she talked about her mother's restful peace and her own grace I got stronger. Playing with the kids and eating a meal at mom and dad's house was health care. Comparing that form of health care to a doctor entering my room and not hearing a word I said because he's thinking of how he made a dot-to-dot with my x-ray that afternoon, I'd rather have the former.

It was bad enough not always being validated as a human, but the oncologists were even more intimidating when they made their rounds traveling as a pack. The ratio was one nearly naked, emotionally spent patient, losing his strength and savings, to six white-cloaked physicians with pocket protectors and stethoscopes surrounding the bed and asking if everything's all right. The attending doctor was flanked by five intern/bouncers who were required by law to be even less animated than himself. It created the ominous feeling of a Senate hearing and, while hoping they'd save my life, I wanted them out of there.

My goal was to get someone in the group to laugh or at least break a smile. Not a huge one, but it was my statement that the other patients and I were more than just bed occupants. I wasn't afraid to speak up, yet I was still intimidated by the medical Mafia. How did other, less confident people handle the pressure? How would my father, who had his cancer five years after I did, have handled it? Fortunately he had expert hospice care during his last days. But I can't imagine how he would have felt at the mercy of a swarm of white coats and not truly being able to understand what was going on. His anxiety would have been tripled beyond the awful fear of dying.

Traveling together, the doctors could control any situation or answer and question of even the most confident patient. But as I witnessed, if you get one of those guys alone and say the right thing, it's like a wolf cub cut off from the pack. I don't mean it maliciously, but it was a pleasure watching one of my new roommates keep a doctor on the ropes. Although I never spoke to the man, I likened him to Rex, my first roommate, in that he had plenty of other physical ailments and cancer as well. What I remembered most about him, though I can't remember his name, was that he was a quiet and unassuming elderly gentleman with what appeared to be a severe skin condition. He wasn't the type I would have thought capable of sending a doctor packing.

I tried not to make too much of his condition because, although it looked severe to me, it's possible he and his family felt it wasn't a problem. Regardless of any of his afflictions, he was a kindly and gentle-voiced man. His family came in, two or three at a time, gathered at the side of his bed and talked as if exchanging small town news; "Mavis finally got the new blower for her furnace so she doesn't have to stay with Aunt Lolly anymore." His guests would run off daily accounts as if to keep my roommate abreast of the goings on outside his room. "So Sherry brought Bert to the boat show. You know 'cause Bert can't drive on account of his hip … " And that fellow listened patiently, occasionally chiming in with an "Oh" or an empathetic "Mmm."

One day the curtain between our sides of the room was half open as I was trying to force myself to get some sleep. My eyes were half at rest so they looked closed but were open just slightly, allowing me to look about the room.

In through the door entered a young physician to speak with my roommate. The room was dark gray, the kind where even if the shades are closed in the daytime the sun still gets through. Because my roommate had the light on above his bed, I got a good view of all that went on. The doctor pulled up a chair and sat right next to the man's bed.

"Tomorrow morning we would like to have some of the fellow doctors and interns come in and take a look at your stomach."

The man didn't respond and just looked politely at the doctor.

"Your case is extremely unusual and we'd like some of the newer interns to get a look at the twisting structure it's taken on."

With a polite tone, the man finally spoke up. "I'm sorry. I don't think I would like them all coming in here."

Since I'd only seen the condition that ran up and down his back, which seemed totally separate to what they were discussing, I could hardly believe he had a whole other problem with his stomach as well. The doctor was taken off his game by the man's response but pressed on.

"We really think it would be a benefit to all of us if we had a more extensive look at it."

Again the gentleman simply replied, "I'm sorry. I really don't want my body to be viewed like that. I don't think I would feel comfortable."

"It would be an excellent opportunity for us to learn something, especially the younger doctors who've never seen this kind of thing."

"I don't think so. I'd rather my body not be viewed like that."

The doctor looked up and around for back-up, waiting for

another doctor to step in and say, "I agree. It would be good for all humanity if you let us see your stomach."

The doctor said again, "I'm certain it would be helpful to all of us."

"No. I'm sorry. I wouldn't feel comfortable."

An awkward pause passed.

Finally conceding, the doctor said, "Okay. Please let us know if you change your mind. The staff will be on the floor tomorrow morning."

"Thank you," the man replied, maintaining his kind voice.

The doctor got up and left the room. Because I don't use this kind of language I can't repeat exactly what the gentleman said, but anyone would get the point. After his bout of exemplary patience the man waited a beat and, just before the doctor had crossed the threshold, in an exasperated, fed-up tone, he said "F***ing kids."

I kept my eyes at half mast. I didn't want him to see me peering in on the episode, but in my head, as I pretended to sleep, I shouted out an endorsing, "All riiiiiiiight!"

School's Out!

My last day of chemo was November 12th 1992, one day before my 31st birthday. But knowing I was going to be done with chemo for good reminded me of the excitement of the last day of school. If I had books I would have flung them aside. If I hadn't been on crutches I would have ran exuberantly. If I had a teacher I would have kissed her full on the lips and dashed out the door. But I wasn't at school. I was in a sedate, sterile white room, reeking of medicine, with a team of nurses tending to others who *weren't* getting out. No year-books to sign, no erasers to throw. On the outside I acted adult, smiled and said I was sure glad chemo was over. Inside, however, I was as giddy as a kindergartner.

It was only one week earlier that I had walked confidently onto the hospital floor for my last dose of chemo. The sickening smell met me at the elevator like the fellow who greets me with a cart at Target. But knowing it was the last time I had to go through it, I felt more like a visitor than a patient. Instead of thinking, "Why don't they do something about that wretched odor?" I thought, "Gee, what a dreadful smell. I'm sure glad I don't have to come up *here* on a regular basis." I smiled while hobbling on crutches down the hall to the nurses stand. As they checked me in, I felt as if I was only signing up for summer camp. I was a guy with a secret. I didn't want to flaunt it but I felt I was playing the silly game I played as a kid, smugly intoning with peaked eyebrows and a smile, "I know something you don't know … "

My wonderful secret took the edge off of the problems that normally made me roll my eyes and crack a sarcastic joke. "The chemo won't be ready until five tonight? Oh well. I suppose that's the way it goes. Why sure you can take my temperature. You can take my pulse. You can take my blood pressure. You can take me down to old St. Louie. Hey, instead of having me get on the scale, why don't you guess my weight like they do at the fair. Come on. See if you can pick me up, then I'll do you. Whadda ya say?"

For the first time since chemo began, I had the guts to ask for Zofran instead of Attivan. I could have asked for it at any other time, but since it was my last week, I had no fear of taking chances. I was feeling celebratory. I said to my nurses, "This is my last week, what the heck, why not try Zofran again?" After they agreed, we both saw the rewards of the change. My body didn't react to the Zofran and I had only minor spit-ups, as opposed to the voluminous vomiting I did without it.

I had the courage to try nearly anything. After all, it was the last week. "Sure, I'll try Zofran again. Yeah, maybe I can eat a little food. What's that you say? You'd like to smear me with paté, put some cherry tomatoes on my eyes, fill my belly button with cheese whiz and use me as a centerpiece to a catered party? Why not?! It's my last week!"

Throughout chemo, the thought of my treatments nearly being over served as inspiration — but never more so than that last week. If for some reason it didn't end, I hoped I could be just as joyful . Perhaps I was getting out of chemo and cancer was over, but as Gilda Radner's character Roseanne Roseannadanna had often said, "It's always something." Even if I were through with cancer forever, what if I developed back problems, or terrible allergies or acne; would that mean I'd have to wait for those to end before I experienced joy again? If I waited until everything was perfect before I felt joy, then I couldn't expect joy ever while I was alive because, "It's *always* something."

Did I have joy in my life even when cancer wasn't coming to a close? What about sitting on our bedroom floor and talking with Cheryl? What about going to the zoo with Arlene and the kids? What about the deep, natural laugh of David when I told him about my first proctology exam? Not that it was only joy, there was the blood infection, Cheryl's mom, my painful dreams and the horrible feelings my cancer gave to others.

During those times Roseanne Roseannadanna's words could have even been turned up a notch: it's always something *squared*. If cancer was a huge dive into the pile of goo that is life, at least I enjoyed the climb out. That was how my first day was spent, living and re-living my history as a cancer survivor — as a human being. I wasn't even out of chemo yet and I was already looking on it as a memory.

That day I traveled from my earliest memories all the way through diagnosis, surgeries, visits, my time at home, to the show I did at St. Helena's Church the week before. "What?!" I thought to myself. "A show?" It took a while for it to sink in, but the week before I went in for my last chemo, I did a show at my church's Halloween party. What I had hoped for was a guest set at a comedy club. Even though I was bald, thin and pasty white, I knew I could be funny. If the audience got over their pity and the shock, they'd laugh at the jokes I'd written. Part of me realized that if I had done a show looking like a chemo patient, the audience would have been so taken aback that I would have looked like a pathetic version of one of Jerry's kids scoring money in the off season. But the other part wanted to taste the adventure and break all the rules of comedy. Because of the re-break of my leg, and needing to stay on crutches, I never made it into a club. That might be why I forgot about St. Helena's. I was so bent on my first goal, I didn't think of the Halloween party as a real show.

When they asked me to do their party I said, "You've got to be kidding." I'd done shows for them in the past, but during none of those shows did I look like a thin, handicapped Uncle Fester. But, no, they weren't kidding. "Just do some basic juggling," John, our religious education director said, "The kids love that. It's still entertaining." If I had taken the time to size up the situation I probably would have said no. My juggling skills weren't sharp, my timing would certainly be off, and I would look more out of place than Rush Limbaugh in a hip hop club. But I didn't take the time. I mulled it over for a moment then, as I did every time they asked me to perform for children, grudgingly agreed. Maybe deep down I wanted to do it. Maybe I wanted to see if I could still perform. Maybe I thought my look could lend to the ghoulish aura of a Halloween party. Maybe I thought I was getting paid.

Our kids got all dressed up for trick or treating, Matthew as a handlebar-mustached cowboy in black, Dylan as his favorite Nintendo character, a plumber named Mario, and Rachel as a beautiful fairy dressed in pink. Looking back, I wonder why I didn't wear a costume. I had one shot at being shiny white bald on Halloween and I did nothing. Common sense and good natured fun said paint the back of my head black, put a white circle in the middle and go as an eight ball.

After loading up on candy in our own neighborhood, we drove to St. Helena's school. Fortunately I didn't have to worry about getting surprised reactions from the partiers in the gym. Most of the parish was aware of our situation and helped us out in many ways such as cooking food, watching our kids and offering money. And since there had been others in our parish who battled cancer, they didn't look at me as out of the ordinary, which was good. I was past the point where I didn't give my looks a second thought anyhow, and it was even less of a concern within my church. And once I got settled, let our kids run loose and said hi to the other parents dressed as everything from boxers to aliens, I was told my job was to hold the attention of the kids as the other parents put finishing touches on the games and room setups.

I was introduced to about 70 kids and parents gathered on one end of the gym floor and limped, crutches and all, out to center stage. I had visions of Woody Allen's movie "Broadway Danny Rose" in which he played an inept talent agent who booked strangely inappropriate and misfit acts, such as a one armed-juggler and a hypnotist who couldn't get people out of trances. I wondered if I could get his card.

I began by balancing my own crutches on my chin, laying one atop of the other. Then I handed out clubs to the children in the front to throw to me. The fail-safe was letting the kids give me anything they wanted me to juggle. Everything including a football helmet, a trick or treat bag, one piece of candy and an assortment of shoes passed through my hands. If I was smart I would have let that routine be the entire show because the kids never tired of seeing different objects juggled. It was as if they'd say, "Well, you've done a ball, a pair of pants and a pogo stick," then look around frantically, "but you haven't done the record player yet." I was happy to accommodate them, but I also juggled five clubs just to show myself I could do it. As far as the kids were concerned, though, all I had to do was make a funny noise while juggling anything and they'd consider it entertaining.

To get the adults laughing I heckled myself throughout the entire show, pointing out how ridiculous the show must look. For instance, once I even stopped juggling, put down my props and said, "I feel like half the kids here are thinking, 'What's next? A quadriplegic mime?' And the other half are turning to their parents saying, 'Mommy mommy, give him some money and make him stop!'" How could everyone not be thinking I looked strange? Joking about it diffused the uneasiness and helped the parents laugh too.

Although I'm usually my own harshest critic, considering all the oddities, it was a pretty good show. There was plenty of laughter from the adults, the kids were having fun and I was juggling better than I thought I could. But once it was over I hardly gave it another thought because I was more focused on the chemo ahead of me than on the accomplishment behind me. Long after the show, after I was back in chemo with time to think, it hit me — not only had I juggled, I had performed. Without even realizing it I had reached my loftiest goal.

When I first started my treatments I performed without props, using material on friends and family. That was nice and made me feel human but I asked for more. I wanted to juggle, and I did, better than I ever thought I would, with Bryan at the lake. Besides Cheryl loving me so completely, that was the best feeling I had during chemo. And yet I wanted more. I didn't want to just juggle, I wanted to juggle on stage again. And there I was, before my self-imposed time limit expired, on stage at St. Helena's performing for my own parish. I had gotten my wish. Unfortunately, after traveling all that way, after realizing all those goals, it still wasn't enough. Not to be indignant or take my life-changing experience for granted, but I wanted to juggle again for real — make my living on stage again and do comedy about my cancer. I wouldn't know for several more months whether I could perform or not, but I knew more than ever that I wanted to try.

The summer vacation before my last chemo hook-up was almost over. The day flew by in a whirlwind of daydreams and real dreams. I had almost forgotten the reason I was back in the hospital and that an entire week in chemo, even with Zofran, is still a long time. With only a couple hours remaining before the chemicals were ready, I prepared for the mucky business of getting *through* the week. If the end of my experience was comparable to the last day of school, then chemo was the Neanderthal school yard bully making the rounds to ensure that he had beaten up everyone in his class before the school year was up. After finally getting hooked up to the IV, Zofran played the role of the gym teacher watching out his window to make sure the school bully, chemo, didn't get too far out of hand. Because of the Zofran, nausea and pain were minimal. They still existed though and, without Attivan, I had all day everyday to think about it. That posed a strange dilemma. What would I rather do, not feel as sick but be fully awake for an entire week or be sick as a new sailor in a storm and not remember a thing? I opted for staying awake.

With the extra time I got a few more chances to chat with the people who had a hands-on part in saving my life — the nurses. During the six previous weeks, the nurses and I had talked about everything from comedy to family to money to health care. But psychologically, knowing I was there to be treated left a thin veneer of medicine over many of our conversations. For whatever the reason, during the last week I felt there was an unconscious shift in our conversation. It was easier for them to ask, "So now what are you going to do?" It became just a little more personal, a little more emotional — like all of a sudden we were peers. That was the perk in my relationship with the nurses; I made friends. We don't see each other regularly or anything, some I haven't seen since, but I consider every nurse who spent time in my convalescence a friend — whereas, except my complete trust in Dr. Thompson, I consider most of the doctors as rich uncles who've already written me out of their wills.

Unfortunately, the fun, silly and frequent talks I remembered having with my nurses were while I was on Attivan. Back then we'd talk for a while, then I'd zonk out for a couple hours only to find them back in my room so we could talk again. What a surprise it was to realize that they didn't hang around my room all day. They spent most of their days doing their work and dealing with all the patients on the floor. And that didn't fit into my plans for my last week. The same formula held true for visits. The reason it seemed like I had visitors all day long was because Attivan helped blend one visit into another. Without Attivan I had to wait hours, sometimes a whole day, for someone to visit me. Without the round-the-clock attention I was used to, I turned again to my shiny

19" friend bolted up in the hospital room corner.

When I had watched TV while I was drugged up, it was just noise, a distraction. I didn't take it seriously and, in my condition, didn't feel as if I was really watching it. I was burning time until I slept again. I had berated the trash TV I saw and shook my head in wonder, but, without the drugs, I wasn't just commenting from a distance, I was a participant. The next time that I caught myself tuned into a trashy daytime show, gaping wide-eyed at some terrible topic such as "Sex Slaves for Hire and the Midgets Who Love Them," I was like an old woman aghast, an open hand on my chest and the other fanning my face and gasping, "Why I *never*!" I felt like I had just been woken up while sleepwalking through the middle of downtown naked. "Oh my God, what am I doing here? Is there anyone watching?"

I turned off the TV and didn't watch another talk show for the rest of my stay. Occasionally I watched a little PBS. I had thought for years that "Sesame Street," while also being a good penance for watching the crummy junk I did, qualified as one of the best and most watchable shows on television. It was better than half of what was on prime time. They could replace Tim Allen of the hit series "Home Improvement" with Bert, of Bert and Ernie, and audiences would scarcely notice the difference. Heck, put Ernie in as that guy on the other side of the fence and ratings would go through the roof.

Without the TV or people filling up my room, I had little left to rely on. Chemo had fried me so badly I didn't have ideas to write in my book anymore. It was only the second day and the week already felt long. I had such confidence the day before when I entered chemo, but anxiety and fatigue had set in and I was beginning to feel sorry for myself. Attivan had kept me zoning in and out enough that I usually forgot to mope like that, but it wouldn't that way for my last week of chemo. With no outside influences to busy me and a clear mind for the entire 168 hours, I could hardly think of anything to do *but* feel sorry for myself.

How ironic that, not only was I so upbeat a day and half earlier, but that last week was the only time I shouldn't have had to feel sorry for myself. Everything was going right. I was almost done. I was on Zofran. I had even done a show for goodness sakes, so what more did I want? I had already answered that question though. I wanted my performing days back, to not be in the hospital anymore. I wanted the nearly a year of my life back, without the misdiagnoses, without the operations and broken leg, without the chemo and without the cancer. I wanted to be normal like everyone else.

I was frustrated. My feelings were like oil and water together in the same bowl because at the same time I was feeling sorry for myself, I was also ashamed for feeling that way — ashamed for feeling what I went through was any more difficult than anyone else's life, than any of the other eight million cancer survivors, than anyone who comes from a troubled home, from my own deaf parents' lives. Who was I to complain?

I couldn't get out of my mind all the people that surrounded me throughout my ordeal. I remember Cheryl watching me clean my Hickman, Dave bringing me soup, and Bryan's brother, Barry, sending me a couple delightfully esoteric notes. After the Minneapolis newspaper ran an article about a huge benefit that Bill Arnold put together for our family, people we didn't even know treated us as if we were special. Both Cheryl and I thought, "There's no way we can live up to this." We thought we were just ordinary people in an extraordinary circumstance. I thanked them, but I also felt bad because they didn't fully know me. They never saw me yelling at my kids or being stubborn to Cheryl, being too self involved with my own projects, neglecting the family and being self-centered as performers tend to be. They didn't know me, but still they poured out their hearts in sweetness, sincerity and kindness to help us get by. How ironic that I lived most of my childhood alone and now I had more people caring about me than I knew what to do with.

I wished I could have invited every one of those people over to sit and talk. The love poem I wrote for my family, I realized, was for them as well and for anyone who had the desire to give or receive love. It wasn't possible, but I wanted to share my life with them — the good and the bad — and they could share theirs with me. I wanted to give something to so many of the people who had thought about me, Cheryl and the kids. But my social inadequacy, which proved to be my cruelest characteristic, kept me numb. The impoliteness I fought for as a child, which included not sending thank-you or good-will notes, had become my plague as an adult. If ever I needed those skills it was right then sitting in my hospital bed. Even now, years past chemo, I have written thank-yous to barely half of those who extended their grace.

From the very beginning to the last week, with each passing moment of chemo, my humility grew, yet each time I failed to act upon it. The clearest evidence was my relationship with my great-aunt Catherine. She was my pain-buddy throughout all the surgeries and chemo. At 87 years old, Catherine was in the midst of the worst time of her life, medically speaking. She suffered from severe pain on the heel of her foot, a broken hip from a fall, had lost her desire to eat and, because of her limited ability to care for herself, lost desire for most everything other than her two surviving sisters.

Known as "Toots" by close family members, Catherine would call me on occasion and we'd talk about our experiences. It always astounded me at how she genuinely thought what I was going through was so awful, even as she told me of her own experiences that had me saying, "I can't believe what you've gone through." It was ironic because, even as we each told terrible stories of pain, we both would laugh. Sometimes I'd make a joke or exaggerate my diagnosis like the time I told her, "The new bone in my leg runs on Duracell batteries." Other times we got to the point where our lives seemed so ludicrous that they couldn't possibly get worse, and we'd laugh because there was nothing else to do.

I remember that every time we talked she would say the same thing. In her kindly, weathered voice, between the stories of what she was going through and trying to encourage me, she always said, matter of factly, "Old age is Hell." It might well be but Aunt Catherine was heaven.

I remember visiting Catherine and her sisters Marie and Agnes at her home in White Bear Lake, Cheryl and I accompanying my parents and Arlene. Seeing them all together, Cheryl and I loved their incredible spirits. Their love of each other, their sense of humor and deep memories were shining examples of growing old. They were all simply beautiful people, yet in her need when old age was not in her favor, when she was in pain, not once did I visit Catherine on my own. I made a couple of calls but it was she who initiated most of them. I made many plans but never fulfilled them. Sure I wanted to perform again, wanted to get my life back on track, wanted to embrace joy every second of existence, but did that mean I couldn't make time for others — especially those I loved and who were in need? I once accompanied my mother who always made it a point to visit Catherine as well as her sisters. I told myself I had to visit her more often, but in the five years since the joyful visit with her sisters until Aunt Catherine's death in 1994, I only visited her one more time, tagging along with my parents.

Aunt Catherine and my mother came from the old school that said you were obligated to make every effort to visit, call or write. I, sadly, had come from the new progressive school of self-justification that said, "I really *should* stay in touch but if I don't at least I know I tried." It is a school of considerably less honor.

I don't know how many days I spent under that cloud of shame. But however many it was, I don't think it will ever go away because I allowed it to happen and I can't take any of it back: I didn't visit Catherine, I didn't reply to all who sent their prayers, so even when my life is filled with joy, I will always be responsible for that. Perhaps God will give me another chance someday to act and I hope I will answer the call.

My sorrow must have lasted a couple of days or more because I soon found myself near the end of the week. By that time, because of sad feelings and long days, my demeanor had somehow changed from, "Hey! It's my last week!" to "Two more stinking days and I'll be done." I could have been counting days, hours and minutes from the moment chemo started; I'm sure some patients did. But I began when the end was so close I could taste it. Unfortunately, it tasted lousy so, since I didn't have a roommate, I closed my door, left the lights off and shut the curtain.

I didn't have any more visitors which was the perfect accompaniment for my decision to sulk for the rest of the week. Then, the next day, disrupting my bad attitude, a young doctor came in saying he needed to give me a physical. "What?!" I thought, "I get out tomorrow. Why in the world would it be imperative that you come in now to see if my bones are bending the right way?" But the only way I communicated my rage was with a heavy sigh, saying, "Oh, okay."

I didn't trust him from the moment he walked in the room. He had wavy dark red hair, a pasty complexion and shifty eyes, although the main reason I didn't trust him was probably because of his white lab coat and clipboard. I hadn't met or seen him before and was offended that he even asked me to get up. Also he was a little more thorough than I liked, looking at places on my body *I've* never even seen before. Afterwards I planned to go to the nurses station and say, "I really didn't like the way Dr. Slayton gave me a physical. I wasn't ready for it and he easily could've scheduled it for a later time." Only I was deathly afraid the nurses were going to say, "Um, sorry but there is no Dr. Slayton that works here."

There seemed to be a quota of miserable things I had to feel before chemo was finished. First there was my anxiousness to leave, then my self-pity and shame. Also there was the annoying physical, and I'd just had two of the worst night's sleeps I'd had in years. The quota was finally filled when my first and only room-mate of the week checked in on the very day I was leaving. At seven a.m. I heard him talking comfortably and confidently, like a chemo veteran, with the nurses and his girlfriend. All of them talked loudly or at least they weren't using, as we say at the Burton home, their "quiet voices." They couldn't have known I wanted to sleep though. They were speaking in their regular voices, assuming everyone in the hospital must be up pretty early, considering the window shades don't keep the light out, the nurses station was bustling and there was a young woman who went into every room taking blood samples by seven. But that doesn't take into account a young fellow who was up until five a.m. for the past couple of nights. I didn't want to be angry about it though because there were worse things that I could have awakened me. "At least," I thought, "the doctor's not coming in and saying, 'Sorry, Scott, we made a mistake. We've been giving you the wrong chemo and would like to start over with some new stuff. Okay?" Things weren't that bad after all.

"I can cope with this," I thought. "I'm getting out today. He's coming *in* for chemo for goodness sake's. He's the one who should be cranky. I really shouldn't mind. He sounds like a nice guy. I'll be fine as long as he doesn't start a convers ..."

"Hi, how you doin'."

Quoting Homer Simpson, my brain shouted, "Du-oh."

The last thing I wanted to do was talk. But then I thought, "Maybe all of this is a test." I had decided way back, when I was first diagnosed, that I would happily give myself to, or at least talk with, any fellow survivor who needed my time. Although I have trouble initiating I knew I could give when asked, especially to another cancer survivor. In spirit of Aunt Catherine, I replied, "Pretty good. I'm getting out today. How are you?"

It was wonderful. I had spent the whole week in self-absorption, which was the exact opposite of how I wanted to deal with cancer, when all it took was one fellow patient to burst into my room and talk to me when I least wanted to. He saved me from myself. It was like the buddy system we used as kids at the lake. For all I know the nurses had seen how surly and depressed I was and put that guy in my room on purpose. I thought I knew it all, that I had my system down for handling cancer — pay attention, embrace those around me and, whether it be filled with joy or pain, love my life. By the end of that week, I forgot the most elemental part of my plan: I needed to communicate.

So we talked. And, just as the most wonderful moments can happen when you least expect them, some of the best conversations can begin with the simple words, "Hi, how you doin'." Unfortunately our talk wasn't one of them. We talked about our cancers. He was indeed a veteran and was fighting cancer for a second time. He was also a big comedy fan, so I told him inside stories of the local comedy scene and a little about the national scene. Because I was so tired, I didn't want the conversation to go on, yet I was thankful to have it and not focus on myself.

But what I remembered most of my last week wasn't our talk. It wasn't even that I was done with chemo for good. The moment I will always remember best was when I finally saw my roommate.

Death is known as the great equalizer, but I was witness to chemo being a close second. Chemo strips the body of every stitch of hair, leaving the face almost featureless. And that was what I saw when my roommate got up, passed my curtain and looked directly at me. He was skin bald, lacking eyebrows, eye lashes and all facial hair.

He stood poised in his blue hospital gown when we caught each other's eyes. I was struck numb and silent staring at him and he may have felt the same looking at me. Seeing this man who had lost all the characteristics of his face, I had to feel my arms and chest to make sure I was still in my own hospital bed.

As I gazed eerily at him I couldn't help but think, "That's me!"

Taking My Act On The Road

Part of me would always remain in chemo. The fact that I had been there meant it would always be a part of me. Not intending to steal any thunder from Tom Joad, I would be there in the face of every patient that remained on Masonic 3, in the face of every other person diagnosed with cancer. It was not only the conversation I had with my last roommate that would bring me back to chemo, but the conversations I had with my nurses throughout the week and every conversation I will have with anyone who understands survivorship.

That was how cancer affected me most, by imbedding itself into the rest of my life. Like when my father passed away and Cheryl wasn't sure how I was handling it because I wasn't crying and didn't seem outwardly shaken. Others asking me how I was taking his passing made me question myself as to whether I was missing out on something. Would it hit me all at once? Was I finally going to realize he was gone and hurt deeply because I didn't recognize it? The way I handled it was to accept that his death forever became a part of who I was. A few weeks after his death, I watched my comic friend Colleen talk about her dad during her act and it made me think like I had never done before while watching comedy. "*My dad has died,*" I thought while watching, almost as if I was conversing with her. "*He's gone and I loved him, but I don't get to see him now.*" After the show I still wanted to talk with her about it, tell her stories about my dad like she did about hers. His illness and death would forever be a part of my history and I would live it over and over. Chemo was the same. I will always go back because, like every moment I have lived, it defined who and what I was and that couldn't be taken away.

On the metaphysical and psychological side, I accepted that I would always be in — or a part of — chemo and was even proud of it. On the purely physical side, however, I knew I was going home. Regardless of how sour I'd grown throughout the week, for the last hour or so I sat watching the chemo bag empty as I bounced quietly on my bed like a child with autism rocks back and forth. Since it took an hour for what seemed like mere ounces of liquid to drain out of the bag, I grew eager thinking the IV was going to beep at any moment signaling the chemo was gone. I thought it was purely academic since the amount of chemo in the bag was hardly anymore than I could spit. But the IV refused to beep until the very last drop was gone.

Secretly I hoped they made concessions for the last day of chemo. I thought the nurse would come in and, as I looked pleadingly into her eyes, she'd say like a cop forgiving a speeder, "Aw, what the heck. Unhook yourself and get outta here." That should be a standard service provided for one's last day, I thought. In my opinion, one of the best feelings in life discovering, when faced with something I dreaded, that I didn't have to do the dreadful thing after all — like waking up after a snowstorm and finding the sidewalk already shoveled. And what better thing to miss out on than chemo? A "Get Out Of Chemo Free" card, time off for good behavior, that's what I was looking for. Sadly, they had no such program.

Without the option of early parole, I did little but stare at the dwindling IV bag. Like a kid watches his mother bake brownies, like a lion watches a herd of antelope, like a cop guards a doughnut shop, I stared at that bag. I found myself getting enraged at the indifferent machine. "Beep, blast you. Beep!" My mind wandered, wishing I could throw my voice or make the right noise to simulate the beep. Perhaps channeling would work or the power of telekinesis. I wanted to just start beeping myself at the top of my lungs in high-pitched tones, "Beeeeeeeep. Beep beep beep." I knew that couldn't possibly work after playing out the scene in my head: The nurse comes running in and checks over the IV stand.

"Well, I can't figure out why it beeped. There's still a little chemo left in here."

I sound off again, "Beep beep beep beep beep."

The nurse turns to me, "You did that."

"Did what?"

"You just beeped. It wasn't your chemo."

"I didn't beep. Why would *I* beep? It's the bag. It's empty. Check it."

She turns to look at the bag and I seize the opportunity, "Beep beep."

She rounds on me with Twilight Zone anxiety, "That was *you!*"

"What do you mean? Didn't you hear it? That was the bag," I claim innocently. She keeps leering at me suspiciously. "Really," I insist.

Her eyes stay on me as she slowly turns her head toward the chemo. "Really!" I repeat. Finally, she fakes a look at the bag, then snaps her head back toward me.

"Beeeeeeep."

"Hah! I caught you."

"No you didn't."

"Okay, I'm outta here. Let me know when your bag *really* empties. Or, on second thought, don't."

So there I sat, for the first time in my life, envying ventriloquists.

The last hour in chemo seemed almost as long as the seven months I'd already spent. It was both hard and not hard waiting — a combination of, "Well, I've waited *this* long …" and "If I spend another second here I'm going to lose it." But when it finally ended, when the IV finally beeped, it was the most surreal moment of my life. I couldn't believe my ears. Cancer immediately became part of my past and no longer my present. I was no longer a patient, I was a tourist.

"Free at last, free at last. Thank God Almighty, I'm free at last." Because I knew I was never going back, it felt special to walk without the IV attached. I looked at my room differently. I took pictures. I never said it but I kept thinking in disbelief, "This is really it!? I can go home? I'm done?!" After signing out, saying my good-byes and stepping out the front door of Masonic 3, I could almost feel hair growing right there and then.

The rest of the evening went quickly. I remember my dad picking me up and bringing me to my parents' house. The kids were there all hyped up and silly and Arlene met me with a three foot round mylar balloon, which the kids popped within the first 15 minutes. When that happened, I beamed and said, "It's nice to know they still got it!" Arlene also gave me a little troll doll with pink hair that stuck straight up like Don King's. On the doll she fashioned a little doctor's mask and a white smock with the word *chemo* written inside a red circle with a slash through it. Although the medical staff gave me the screw they'd used to hold the rod in place while it was in my thigh bone, the doll instantly became my favorite chemo souvenir. I sat down at the kitchen table and stretched out to relax and chat with the family as I had done for over half of my life. Holding up my forearm I showed my mom the one last remaining hair on my body and said, "I told you I wouldn't lose all my hair."

I don't remember how long we stayed or what else we talked about. I don't remember Cheryl, the kids and I packing up to go home or going to bed that night. What I remember most, because it wasn't just that night but for days following, was the smile on Cheryl's face. Her smile, her grace, would remain with me just like chemo and just like my father. She was happy for me being done, but her smile said she, too, was free — from a job perhaps harder than mine. As with me, a weight had been lifted from her and she was as light as air, ethereal, happy and giddy. Her smile that day was as full and innocent as a child's, and her beaming face and the deep hug we shared signaled both the end and the beginning of an incredible journey.

For days after going home, every waking moment was like rebirth. Throughout the days when our paths crossed, when I stopped to watch her read to the children, when we talked in the kitchen, the looks we gave each other were so knowing we almost wanted to break out laughing. It was an in-joke we could share forever. On the small rug in front of our living room couch, playing with race cars and Brio train tracks, saying prayers at night, we shared the joke with the kids. The joke was, "Daddy's alive!" They didn't get it, but they will someday.

The happy joke for all of us is that we're alive. We're all set on this planet to try and figure out our lives, and somewhere up in heaven, the angels are watching it like a TV sitcom. The joke is everywhere, in the beginning and the end, the happy and sad, the pain and ecstasy, the every extreme between reality and make-believe. For Cheryl and me, the joke had been with us forever; that's how good of a joke it was. Although we often take it for granted, it was a pure taste of life and was still wet on our lips. The taste was what God meant when he said he was the Alpha and the Omega — that life is everywere. I knew that what we were experiencing was only a fraction of what life truly was, but in that mere taste we shared God's joke. As a comic, I've never heard a better one.

Even though I couldn't always live life that fully, I now understood that I had known what I was going to do with my life all along. I must have just been pretending when I said I wasn't sure what I would do after cancer. Even when my greatest concern was whether I would juggle again, I was wasting my time fretting because there was no doubt that, somehow, I would again perform. If I had lost my leg, I would have bought an appropriate sized stool to prop myself up to juggle, or I would have juggled on my back. My show was all I knew how to do, and though I convinced everyone I would be just as happy with a straight job, I knew I was going to do it even if it meant only having a three minute spot on Open Stage Night every Monday.

Yet I wouldn't have been satisfied only doing open stages. I wanted to be a working comic who could make the cancer experience funny. In the same way I created my juggling show, I worked out material whenever I could and then tried it out at an open stage or during a guest set on the weekend show. Fortunately I had ten years of previous stage experience to fall back on because it was a slow process. From the first moment I mentioned cancer on stage, the audience froze-up, looked around and checked their ticket stubs to see if they were at a fund raiser. Getting them to laugh, even getting them to loosen up, was going to be a lot harder than I thought.

The audience having trouble with the material, though, was my own fault. The jokes I used were lines a fellow cancer survivor might find interesting but that a paying comedy club crowd didn't find funny because they couldn't relate. "Cancer," I said during one of my first times back on stage, "isn't something we have to fear. It's being attacked with such technology that, someday, having cancer is going to be no worse than a 24 hour fever." Pretending I was pitching a commercial, I finished the joke with, "For the minor aches and pains of cancer, try new *Chemo-riffic*. It costs less than the other brands and now has a fresh minty flavor." Occasionally it got a small laugh, but most audiences not only weren't prepared to hear that kind of joke, they didn't get it either. I also tried a joke about chemo being an effective weight-loss plan. Jenny Craig's new slogan would be "Lose all the weight you can vomit up." This one went over even worse than the other because it was gross too.

While trying so hard to make cancer funny, I forgot the key element of good comedy — telling the truth. Maybe it's stretching the truth, maybe it's what you believe is the truth or what you expect to be the truth, but good comedy is usually just revealing one's life. Instead of trying to be clever, why wasn't I telling my story? Cancer, I reasoned, was simply part of my life. And, along with everything else that it is, life *is* funny. Therefore, cancer, as part of my life, is funny too. So if I could, I wanted to share God's joke.

That was when I went on stage and told the truth. I told the audience what chemo was like for me. "Chemo was like a pregnancy," I said. At that point a few women pricked up their ears. "I know because my wife and I have three kids — and those were all pregnancies." They laughed and I halted for a moment, realizing they were paying closer attention because the joke wasn't only about cancer. It was about my life. "My wife and I went through the exact same things." I continued. "Like her, I lost my body shape. I was tired all of the time and, on any given day, I could vomit twice my body weight." The audience tittered. Then I threw in, "So I went through the exact same thing my wife did. Only I didn't get a prize." It was a better laugh than before — more real. But I still felt I could be more descriptive. I finally started using the potent and humorous line I had told everybody who visited me since the week I'd lost all my hair. "People think when you go through chemo you go bald. And that's not true. You don't go bald, you go … hairless. I realized after a few months that I no longer qualified as a mammal." That brought out a good laugh, an identifiable one. I had finally meshed the truth of my story with a good joke.

Thinking I had momentum, I worked up more pieces that told my cancer story in a way that kept audiences at ease. I knew there would always be a little discomfort in even mentioning cancer, but if they then laughed about it, I was both making them comfortable and dispelling some of the fear and mystique of cancer. So I made it a point to mention my medical history in every show. It was only April of '93 but I was so eager that, although my hair had scarcely grown back, I thought I could pull off cancer material anywhere. So I threw my story into my first non-comedy club private show — my first paid show after cancer. It was a country club in the upscale suburb of Wayzata. And although the rest of my show went well, when I got to the cancer material, the well-dressed, affluent audience simply stared uneasily. It felt terrible. Standing on the small stage with track lighting, gazing into their uncertain eyes, I felt like I had just gotten on stage with a bullhorn and announced, "My name is Scott, I'm with the IRS and this is a group audit." I went on with my material anyway, half expecting one of them to stand up and, representing the well-to-do group, say, "I'm sorry, young man. But we don't *get* cancer here."

That show made me question my cancer material again but I kept doing it. I just was a little more careful who I performed it for. Comedy clubs were okay because people come to listen to whatever you have to say as long as it's funny. But at private parties or corporate meetings, people are, in a sense, inviting me into their homes. I wouldn't walk into someone's cocktail party and say to everyone, "Hey come look at this rude, pulsating purple scar running up and down my leg!" Likewise, I couldn't be invited to do a show and talk about cancer for 15 minutes unless they'd asked me to.

That May I got a new performing opportunity, only I didn't know it. Everything was feeling good and getting better: I was fitting into Cheryl's schedule at home, my leg was growing stronger and I thought my show was nearly back on track. It was about that time I got a call from Jim Van Herke. His deep, business-like voice sounded as if he wasn't in the practice of hiring entertainment or that he was even a veteran comedy patron. But he said there was a group of cancer survivors that met every year on the first Sunday of June and, hearing of what I had gone through the past year and knowing I was an entertainer, he wondered if I was interested in doing a show for them.

I was uncertain at first, wondering even if I fit in with his group. I wasn't yet comfortable referring to myself as a "survivor." I'd used the word because I didn't know a better one, but survivor seemed too lofty a title since I had only done what I had to do to get on with my life. When I heard the word *survivor*, I thought of someone having lived through a gunshot wound or having been mauled by a lion. All I did was have cancer. The only time I felt my life was in danger was during my blood infection; except for that, I didn't think cancer was something I survived.

I thought performing for survivors was a great opportunity to do my cancer material in front of people who understood it, but I was also afraid I might offend someone. "It sure sounds interesting, but I really don't know if I should," I said to Jim. "Do you think anyone would mind if I did jokes about my cancer experience?" "You can do whatever you want to do," he said. "We just think it'd be great if you came down and did ten minutes or whatever you felt like."

I was trying to get assurance from him that people wouldn't loathe me if I talked about cancer. After the experience in Wayzata, I hated the thought of finding out that even fellow survivors didn't think my material was funny. I hemmed and hawed and, after thinking it over a few days, agreed to do the show.

For support Arlene came to the show with me. Just as she loved visiting Aunt Catherine, she was always excited to be in a room where people truly knew what it meant to be alive. I was a little leery. I didn't think I would relate to anyone because I assumed I approached my episode in a more lighthearted way than a roomful of other survivors. Never having been around a large group of survivors I expected the majority of people to be spent from their struggle with cancer. I pictured them depressed, maybe angry, as if they were still going through the emotional stages of diagnosis. I wasn't even certain if the gathering would even be a celebration. Instead, I envisioned a hundred or so weathered and tired people sitting around in chairs, looking at each other saying, "Well, we're not dead *yet*."

My heart completely changed and my eyes opened excitedly when I entered the doors to the registration desk. People were up and about, smiling, laughing and sharing stories. Everyone had name tags with the number of years they'd lived beyond cancer. Most I saw were five to ten years. Then I saw 42 years, 30 years, 37 years. I saw nine months on one tag and that person was smiling, juice drink in hand, talking with one of the many friends she had made at the celebration. It was a roomful of life. I felt at home.

Jim, who sounded like a reluctant volunteer over the phone, was the embodiment of the celebration itself. Like a Grand-Poobah initiating a new member into an Elk's club, he introduced me throughout the room. He was a prime example of a joyful survivor, not only making contact with most of the others in the room, but taking part in their lives as well. As I met each person who shared their stories and asked about mine, I grew excited to do my show. They were my people. Or more correctly, because it was their event, I was their people.

Part of me didn't even need to do a show. I had to because that was the best way I knew how to communicate myself, but I would have had just as good of time talking a swapping stories with everyone in that room. Everyone not only had stories to swap, but they were excited to share them. Arlene was mingling and I was getting ready for my show, going over my jokes sitting at a large, round formica table. Watching the crowd of a couple of hundred, I thought, "Everybody has a story, a worthwhile and embraceable one. It's not just being a cancer survivor. We're *all* survivors, surviving the same thing — life." Just being around them made me comfortable with the word. I was suddenly proud to be a survivor. I wanted to work the thought of everyone having a story into my act but wasn't sure how to fit it into a comedy show. Besides, I wanted to focus on the group at hand. Maybe everyone does have a story and maybe sharing that story is all there is to life, but the group around me and I shared a common story — fiercely unique and individual, yet a common story.

It was a big square room that could have easily doubled as a cafeteria, with thin carpeting covering the floor and bright florescent lighting above. I wasn't sure whether the room was conducive to comedy, let alone trying to get away with cancer jokes in front of cancer patients. Jim went to the front of the room and thanked everyone for being there. He then introduced a local television personality who brought up two other survivors to share their stories, then introduced me.

Up until that point I was mentally flipping coins in my head as to whether I should do cancer material or just juggle. I knew they would love the juggling; just seeing someone juggle like I could after going through a yearlong ordeal would certainly be uplifting to them. I reached the stage and decided to test the waters. "It's a pleasure," I told them, "to work in a room where people truly understand the cancer experience. I try to talk about cancer in all my shows. For example, I do shows at a comedy clubs and I'll talk about cancer there and ... *Man!*" I raised my eyebrows and widened my eyes with surprise and the audience laughed heartily with recognition. They had all experienced talking about cancer to those who didn't know how to handle it, so picturing me doing it in a public forum was a delicious rebuttal for them.

I hadn't even told a joke and they laughed. So I went into all my cancer material which, at the time, lasted only about 10 minutes. The recognition of my story grew with every bit. When I reached the part of no longer qualifying as a mammal the room exploded as if we all finally got God's joke. It was as if that group had never heard anything like it before. Maybe they told cancer jokes between themselves to laugh or heard humorists talk about it, but it was as if they had never seen anyone do stand-up comedy about cancer. I felt so honored to be the one to do it that I was excited about also getting to juggle for them. Allowing me to do my jokes was their gift to me; my juggling show was my gift to them.

The show lasted about a half an hour and afterwards people hung around and talked, sharing more stories. The connection was one of pure human spirit, as after hearing my story, more people came up to share theirs. One large young man who looked like a football player and obviously had a lot of anger about his cancer told Arlene and me as we were buying a shirt from him, "It's been two years and I never thought I would laugh about cancer. Today was the first time."

That statement did it for me. Never would I find anything as fulfilling as performing for other survivors. I will always enjoy doing shows, but that day I learned there was a difference between merely doing shows and performing. Performing is doing a show, but the word also indicates getting a job done, being productive. I had been doing shows all my life but that night, maybe for the first time ever, I *performed*.

At my diagnosis, when I wanted to juggle once more, I never knew it could be this good. In hindsight, I had been performing throughout my experience and didn't even know it, talking with Tony and Rex, sharing Cheryl's grace, laughing with Mary Francis — who had ovarian cancer — at church. What performing also means is communicating with love. Whether I had done it previously in my life or not, I know now I want to perform for the rest of my life, with or without cancer.

The evening's festivities ended with all the survivors forming a long line and parading around the room. It was almost like the bunny hop people do at weddings except we didn't hop and our dance meant something. In a silly way it made a profound connection. Celebrating survival was something available to anyone, but these cancer survivors took the time to recognize and live it.

From the first joke with Dr. Thompson to the last hug at the survivor's celebration, I thought I could make it through cancer with joy, and, for the most part, I did. I learned the hard way that it's easier said than done. Sometimes the pains I had, like the blood infection or the burning in my throat, didn't let me experience the joyful moments when they came, but, even then, I was always aware of the possibility of doing so. Because I trusted in joy all the way through it, I felt as if I had walked away from cancer not that much different from the day I went in. Even though I had my own cancer experience, with my own different problems, I had thought that the struggles of all humans were basically the same. It wasn't until my cancer battle was over, when I mixed with that roomful of survivors, that I saw we all have our own individual stories. Mine is the story of a juggler with cancer who learned to get up after a fall. Along with the others who taught me to celebrate, I am a survivor. I am a performer. And, most importantly, I am alive.

Epilogue

Perhaps I am being indulgent, but as I neared the completion of this book, I knew I wanted to include this piece I had written after my father had passed away. Every story in this books has intended to reflect on the humor that I see in life, the humor that I've tried to keep in my heart. I hope that the reader has gotten a few laughs and smiles in the process and has also seen the humor in their own lives. But I also recognize that there are many kinds of humor. Sometimes the best humor is simply being human. As this story is about my father's death, there are no jokes or laughs. But I believe that there is a profound humor that wove in and out of our lives even as dad was dying. It was the humor of all our lives, of our smiles, laughs and shared moments. It was the humor of humanity.

The following was printed in the St. Paul Pioneer Press on September 3 , 1996:

We buried my father a few weeks ago. A metasticized melanoma had traveled from his leg to his lungs and then to his brain, eventually taking his life. The loss, the sorrow, the not under-standing left the entire family in tears. Our first instinct was to cry and ache. It was a good instinct.

Yet none of us could ignore the fact that his death had to happen sometime. He was 75 and for almost the last decade our family knew it was a matter of counting the years. We saw him with eyes that knew both he and we were getting old, yet there was no way we could know how his death would come.

I was the one who had cancer first. My dad, my whole family, stood by me and we all accepted my cancer as part of life. Regard-less of the disease, our lives were full. When I was told there was a 50/50 chance of it returning, the doctor said it would most likely appear in my lungs. How shocked I was, almost as if there was a mistake, when it reappeared in my father's.

Cancer stripped my father of his capability. When he was no longer being able to throw darts, play golf or communicate in a rational way, our second instinct was to think how cruel death was. But, after my own cancer, sometimes I wonder.

By many standards, my dad's life was uneventful, maybe even boring. He was not an award winner, a traveler or one who got a lot of attention. He was only a simple stock cutter, deaf since infancy, who felt like an outsider all of his life. He scarcely had a childhood in a poor Jewish family, mostly tagging along with his three brothers, feeling uncomfortable because he was only able to communicate by making awkward high-pitched sounds associated with deafness.

Even though he found a new world at the Faribault School for the Deaf where he could relate to others and they to him, show his confidence, and even speak clearer, he was always intimidated by the hearing-dominated world he lived in. He was a decent basketball player, a firstbaseman in kittenball and a better than average boxer, but those were all small parts of his life and didn't help him find comfort as a deaf person at the grocery store or the bank.

I remember him best preparing for work as I got ready for school, silently going about his business, cracking open a two-minute egg and eating it right out of the shell as he read the morning news. Everything he did seemed silent, his job, his manner, his work around the house. Some might say my dad's whole life was silent. Where was his statement, his place, his mark? Yet my dad, in life and death, had attained something most of America will never achieve.

He was true.

Harvey Burton lived life without any pretensions. How many of us can say that? He didn't pretend to be anything he wasn't — he didn't even know *how* to. When he spoke you knew he truly believed every word he said, always remaining simple. Even with his hard upbringing, life owed him nothing. He wanted plenty of things he didn't have, and there was plenty he was sad about, but with hardly another word he accepted it. It was still his life and it must have been okay because he was living it.

Others might question the worth of his life, yet no one can tell me its worth was any less than those considered great. The moment any person looked into his eyes and saw a simple and honest man — a humble man — his greatness was written. The moment you looked to him and knew he was someone you could trust you saw the greatness in being a human being, in being alive. It was a simple greatness. And, if he had it, it must be available to us all.

When we first told him that the melanoma had come back in his lungs, I remember him, flush in the face and slightly teary-eyed, saying, "Well, I guess I'll have to start living life one day at a time." I became teary-eyed myself because that was what he had done all along. That was where *I* learned it from. Though I can't plan to save my life, I've never found it difficult to value each day for what it was because of my father.

As things got worse, it was sad watching him lose what he saw as his manhood. He needed help walking and remembering things. He even got lost once walking alone to the end of our block. We all cried thinking that was the worst thing that could happen to him because, in dad's life, all he really needed was control of his own personhood, his own space, a quiet place to read the paper, a job he can accomplish — but he had lost even that. That was cancer's worst blow.

Yet, like the loss of his youth, he accepted it. He let mom tell him all the things he should be doing when normally he would be busy voicing his own opinion (even when he was wrong). But with wide eyes and a half smile, he'd nod and consent to his wife like a child obeying his mother.

The cancer reached his brain and soon he spent all his day on the couch with the TV on though he couldn't hear the sound or read the captioning. He talked in whispers, much of the time not making understandable sense as he battled with bouts of uncognizance and awareness.

In discomfort he'd make soured faces at us and twist and turn signing that it was over, "finished." He signed in his sleep, his brain living stories and memories as his body died.

Those were the worst moments for us, knowing we were helpless. Taking turns, us six kids would visit mom and dad's house and sit, if only to hold dad's hand, to look into his eyes and let him know we were still with him. It was those times we would see him perk up. How much he loved just seeing his family. Once making the connection, his eyes lit up even brighter than in his younger days. Brighter, lightened as if the unburdening of the worries of his life made him see more clearly how happy he was just to be with his family, just to sit and be alive.

What he achieved in death was perfect humility. It was in his eyes for the briefest of moments, sitting on the couch looking up earnestly, hopefully, his weak hands held outstretched in those of my sister, standing in front of him. A quiet smile of joy and a twinkling in his eye said perhaps that was all he was meant to do in life. That was all that mattered, being a part, listening for another voice, the warm grasp of his own child.

When dad breathed his last breath, the whole family was around his bed at home. Because he couldn't hear us, we all had our hands laid on him in the last few hours as our best way to connect and communicate. And when he died we all lost something we can't explain, a part of ourselves, a part of our family, a part of life.

But something too was gained. We got to be a part ourselves, of another life, of each other once more. We got to share the close-ness we all once had and, together, say goodbye to our father in the kindest way we knew how. It was — and I believe there is such a thing — a good death.

God bless him.